How I Rebuilt My Immune System After M.S.

How I Rebuilt My Immune System After M.S.

✦

And lived a better quality of life

J. L. Wilson, E.A.

iUniverse, Inc.
New York Lincoln Shanghai

How I Rebuilt My Immune System After M.S.
And lived a better quality of life

iUniverse books may be ordered through booksellers or by contacting:

iUniverse
2021 Pine Lake Road, Suite 100
Lincoln, NE 68512
www.iuniverse.com
1-800-Authors (1-800-288-4677)

Because of the dynamic nature of the Internet, any Web addresses
or links contained in this book may have changed
since publication and may no longer be valid.

You should not undertake any diet/exercise regimen recommended in
this book before consulting your personal physician. Neither the author
nor the publisher shall be responsible or liable for any loss or damage
allegedly arising as a consequence of your use or application of any
information or suggestions contained in this book.

ISBN: 978-0-595-44419-9 (pbk)
ISBN: 978-0-595-88748-4 (ebk)

Printed in the United States of America

Contents

IMMUNE SYSTEM BACKGROUND

After accepting a second neurological medical opinion diagnosis of m.s. in 2000, multiple sclerosis appeared devastating. Never had I experienced a major illness in my life of 40 plus years. This was not the end of my life and the good news was that this was not a contagious disease. Fear of spreading what I had to friends or family members was not a secondary worry.

Spurred by my desire for my children and myself to live a better quality of life I took off on a journey in 2004 to seek answers to make this happen. My son, daughter, nephew and niece inspired me the most to translate my miracles into writing. Having observed them grow up, their lifestyles, and friends convinced me that I must do something for generations to come.

Some of my most successful findings that I initially embraced were taken from Dr. Lorraine Day, M.D., Dr. Rovenia Brock, PhD., nutritionist and Author, Reese Dublin. All have written books and Dr. Day has published tapes that I used as part of my initial research and foundation for my approach. All books and tapes were related to health and nutritional issues to get well and live better afterwards. There were other contributing experts and references used in my findings and research. These included Dr. Stuart Berger, M.D., Nutritionist Gladys Lindbergh, Joel Fuhrman, M.D. There were others used in my research but these were the most notable. Some of their findings and material are referenced in this book.

After utilizing Dr. Day's tapes and books and leading author in medical research, Reese Dublin, I discovered the core of a natural approach that soon afterwards successfully got me off all medications. This approach also repaired several other areas of my body functions. These have been confirmed by leading medical professionals. Maintaining regular six month interval check ups with my neurologist, urologist, medical internist, and eye doctor during my transition gave me a comfort level of forward progress.

Each of these professionals cited significant improvement and positive changes in my overall health and their specific areas of expertise. Immediate changes were detected during my first six months of committing to a natural approach. More extensive reading gave me a better understanding about why all of these positive things happened to my body. Also, it showed me that the body has a protector. This protector is called the immune system. We all were born with an immune system that keeps us well if we keep it properly maintained. This was just a bunch of medical terms that I barely understood at first. As I continued my reading and research I knew it was a lot to this immune system.

Some of the most noted and immediate things that told me my immune system had positively changed were:

No cold nor any kind of related medical illness for over eighteen months. This happened despite subjecting myself to extremely cold temperatures outside every day and especially early in the mornings; my digestive system began functioning normal without medications, over the counter and doctor prescribed; my urologist informed me that my enlarged prostate discovered enlarged during my early 20's had noticeably shrunk; colon problems previously treated by doctors had changed positively; my energy level improved significantly to me and others; walking longer distances was less of a problem; I used no medications for previously treated medical conditions; my eyesight problems stabilized; and sleep and rest habits improved noticeably. One doctor even told me to stop using medications he had previously prescribed until further notice and suggested some more exploratory medical testing he wanted to do.

Early in my search for knowledge on how I could successfully improve myself without bad things happening to me (side effects), I accepted a fact that it took certain essential things each day of a person's life to live disease free, get rid of major diseases and remain disease free. I also believed it was God's will to allow such things to happen. Significant and noticeable improvement followed my intense desire to use the essential things each day I believed would allow me to get better. It occurred to me to follow these things each day without compromise.

During my diagnosis with multiple sclerosis, I was told by medical experts it was a disease started by a breakdown of my immune system. I first thought this had a whole lot to do with just my nerves. My daughter straightened me out on this subject by telling me multiple sclerosis affected my central nervous system. This meant my brain, spinal cord and nerves. I said, oh.

But my search for knowledge had just begun. Surfing the internet I found out my daughter was right. The immune system was totally different. Even though I read the information, I still thought I had to find cures for my brain, nerves and spinal cord to get better. Several books and tapes later I chose my approach that began to show positive results.

Never will I forget the many conversations I had with friends and associates about the possible causes of m.s. Modern medicine had no known cure for it. However, the most interesting conversation I had about the immune system came about with one of my best friends. He wondered if all of the playground basketball of 30 plus years caused damage to my spinal system. Entertaining his thoughts I managed to laugh inside at first but even gave his comments further consideration during my research efforts.

So far I have talked a lot about immune system. This big imaginative and mysterious thing that had turned my life upside down was called the immune system. The next few pages show you some graphics on the human immune system and its makeup. This was taken directly from some internet material supplied by the National Institute of Allergy and Infectious Diseases. I am not a medical doctor and that is why I chose not to give you a narrative at this point about the immune system. You have to see the medical experts at this point with your questions, not me.

The remainder of my book shares with you the things I used to successfully rebuild my immune system after being diagnosed with multiple sclerosis or m.s.

NIAID*NetNews*
"Advancing Knowledge, Improving Health"

National Institute of Allergy and Infectious Diseases

The Immune System

- 50 YEARS
- NIAID HOMEPAGE
- INFECTIOUS DISEASES
- IMMUNOLOGIC DISEASES
- AIDS
- THE IMMUNE SYSTEM
- NIAID HISTORY
- NIAID DIRECTORS
- WANT TO KNOW MORE?
- NIAID HOMEPAGE
- NIH HOMEPAGE

- The Body's First Line of Defense
- How the Immune System Works
- Antibodies
- T Cells
- Immune System Process

The Body's First Line of Defense

The immune system is a complex of organs--highly specialized cells and even a circulatory system separate from blood vessels--all of which work together to clear infection from the body.

The organs of the immune system, positioned throughout the body, are called lymphoid organs. The word "lymph" in Greek means a pure, clear stream--an appropriate description considering its appearance and purpose.

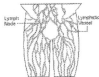

Lymphatic vessels and lymph nodes are the parts of the special circulatory system that carries lymph, a transparent fluid containing white blood cells, chiefly lymphocytes.

Lymphatic vessels form a circulatory system that operates in close partnership with blood circulation.

Lymph bathes the tissues of the body, and the lymphatic vessels collect and move it eventually back into the blood circulation. Lymph nodes dot the network of lymphatic vessels and provide meeting grounds for the immune system cells that defend against invaders. The spleen, at the upper left of the abdomen, is also a staging ground and a place where immune system cells confront foreign microbes.

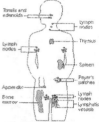

Organs and tissues of the immune system dot the body in a protective network of barriers to infection.

Pockets of lymphoid tissue are in many other locations throughout the body, such as the bone marrow and thymus. Tonsils, adenoids, Peyer's patches, and the appendix are also lymphoid tissues.

Both immune cells and foreign molecules enter the lymph nodes via blood vessels or lymphatic vessels. All immune cells exit the lymphatic system and eventually return to the bloodstream. Once in the bloodstream, lymphocytes are transported to tissues throughout the body, where they act as sentries on the lookout for foreign antigens.

How the Immune System Works

Cells that will grow into the many types of more specialized cells that circulate throughout the immune system are produced in the bone marrow. This nutrient-rich, spongy tissue is found in the center shafts of certain long, flat bones of the body, such as the bones of the pelvis. The cells most relevant for understanding vaccines are the lymphocytes, numbering close to one trillion.

The two major classes of lymphocytes are B cells, which grow to maturity in the bone marrow, and T cells, which mature in the thymus, high in the chest behind the breastbone.

B cells produce antibodies that circulate in the blood and lymph streams and attach to foreign antigens to mark them for destruction by other immune cells.

B cells are part of what is
known as antibody-mediated
or humoral immunity, so
called because the antibodies
circulate in blood and lymph,
which the ancient Greeks
called, the body's "humors."

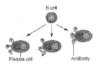

**B cells become plasma cells,
which produce antibodies
when a foreign antigen
triggers the immune
response.**

Certain T cells, which also patrol the blood and lymph for foreign
invaders, can do more than mark the antigens; they attack and
destroy diseased cells they recognize as foreign. T lymphocytes are
responsible for cell-mediated immunity (or cellular immunity). T
cells also orchestrate, regulate and coordinate the overall immune
response. T cells depend on unique cell surface molecules called the
major histocompatibility complex (MHC) to help them recognize
antigen fragments.

Antibodies

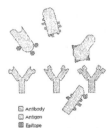

□ Antibody
□ Antigen
▨ Epitope

**Antibodies produced by cells of
the immune system recognize
foreign antigens and mark them
for destruction.**

The antibodies that B
cells produce are basic
templates with a special
region that is highly
specific to target a given
antigen. Much like a car
coming off a production
line, the antibody's frame
remains constant, but
through chemical and
cellular messages, the
immune system selects a
green sedan, a red
convertible or a white
truck to combat this
particular invader.

However, in contrast to cars, the variety of antibodies is very large.
Different antibodies are destined for different purposes. Some coat
the foreign invaders to make them attractive to the circulating
scavenger cells, phagocytes, that will engulf an unwelcome microbe.

When some antibodies combine with antigens, they activate a cascade of nine proteins, known as complement, that have been circulating in inactive form in the blood. Complement forms a partnership with antibodies, once they have reacted with antigen, to help destroy foreign invaders and remove them from the body. Still other types of antibodies block viruses from entering cells.

T Cells

T cells have two major roles in immune defense. Regulatory T cells are essential for orchestrating the response of an elaborate system of different types of immune cells.

Helper T cells, for example, also known as CD4 positive T cells (CD4+ T cells), alert B cells to start making antibodies; they also can activate other T cells and immune system scavenger cells called macrophages and influence which type of antibody is produced.

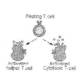

Certain T cells, called CD8 positive T cells (CD8+ T cells), can become killer cells that attack and destroy infected cells. The killer T cells are also called cytotoxic T cells or CTLs (cytotoxic lymphocytes).

T lymphocytes become CD4+ or helper T cells, or they can become CD8+ cells, which in turn can become killer T cells, also called cytotoxic T cells.

Immune system process
Activation of helper T cells

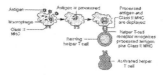

After it engulfs and processes an antigen, the macrophage displays the antigen fragments combined with a Class II MHC protein on the macrophage cell surface. The antigen-protein combination attracts a helper T cell, and promotes its activation.

Activation of cytotoxic T cells

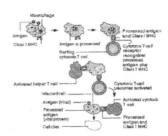

After a macrophage engulfs and processes an antigen, the macrophage displays the antigen fragments combined with a Class I MHC protein on the macrophage cell surface. A receptor on a circulating, resting cytotoxic T cell recognizes the antigen-protein complex and binds to it. The binding process and a helper T cell activate the cytotoxic T cell so that it can attack and destroy the diseased cell.

Activation of B cells to make antibody

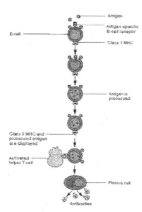

A B cell uses one of its receptors to bind to its matching antigen, which the B cell engulfs and processes. The B cell then displays a piece of the antigen, bound to a Class II MHC protein, on the cell surface. This whole complex then binds to an activated helper T cell. This binding process stimulates the transformation of the B cell into an antibody-secreting plasma cell.

Top of Page

Last updated September 25, 2003 (alt)

1

WALT'S FIRST PRESCRIPTION-EXERCISE

Physical fitness was always a valuable part of my life. As a youngster in high school, oftentimes when idle and not studying assignments I ran the countryside roads alone for miles. I participated in basketball and made it as far as the varsity b team in high school.

You must understand that we didn't have a football program in the county during my middle and high school years. Many of our county and neighboring athletes made it to collegiate and pro levels.

I grew up in a housing project with one such person. This person's entire family including grandparents, sisters, brothers and first cousins lived in three different units. This man and his son made it to the NBA. My level of play never exceeded playground caliber compared to most of the people in my community.

My real sport was baseball. Left handed from birth, my high school baseball coach was determined to make me a left handed ace. I continued this in college but threw my arm away because I didn't use my legs. My collegiate coaches knew it was knee problems but neither my coaches nor I had any suspicion that m.s. may have played its part on my knees early.

Playing basketball vigorously continued during my adulthood until my early forties. After playing, I coached youth basketball until the Atlanta Olympics ended in 1996. Basketball and baseball remained my favorite sports pastimes during adulthood. I picked up golf in the 1980's from job associates and became pretty good at it. This was practically a part-time job because of my positions with a fortune 100 company for years. A noticeable limp began chasing me first in my right leg then switched to my left during my early morning run/walks with my family. This was unusual and I cautiously watched this limp on my own for a couple of months without doing anything about it except to continue walking and no more running. There was no pain associated with the limp, just a limp which made me appear to have pain.

As my approach did not appear to be doing any good, I sought the services of my old collegiate baseball trainer. Walter Smith (Walt). Walt was still in this profession between Morris Brown College and Georgia Tech. Walt immediately began to work with me and put me on a weight resistance training program.

Walt worked with me at times that no other human being could imagine. Most all of the former athletes from my alma mater knew of Walt's total commitment to his profession. This is why I sought Walt after all this time. He didn't let me down.

Walt called the program he initially placed me on a rehab program for injured athletes. He treated me just like that too. I worked out with active collegiate athletes who were pursuing their degrees and dreams of becoming professional athletes. This was fun and not at all awkward like I thought it would be. After all I was nearly twice the age of most of the active athletes. However, they were very disciplined, patient and respectful young people. They were certainly clones of Walt.

At one of the two institutions Walt regularly treated me, I was able to share lockers with one of the rising baseball stars that landed in the Cincinnati Reds organization. This young man had the same characteristics as every other person that I had been associated with who eventually achieved pro status in their profession. This young man was dedicated, humble, trusted in God and had a gentle (peaceful) spirit, almost Christ like. These traits caused me to take special notice and I made sure I emulated these characteristics as close as I could in my approach to the tasks Walt had given me. This became natural. Walt's work ethics, vision and style quickly made me a believer in the hope of getting better with sports medicine. Dedication quickly rushed in and remained with me in every thing I did. I did not even know I had attained a total commitment to using the things Walt had shown me on a daily basis the rest of my life.

The beginning stage of Walt's rehab program called pre-exercise routines included heat with towels and stretches. Next weight resistant exercises were carefully chosen by Walt and added as he watched my responses to various exercises and equipment. Walt tried bicycling and that was too strenuous for me initially because my leg muscles appeared so weak to him. He tested my total conditioning by trying various other routines including steps on a stool he had built for his student athletes, leg weights on Olympic style benches, and stretch band routines. I didn't have a clue what he was doing initially.

After a couple of sessions the program Walt placed me on called for interval training every other day for maximum three days per week. The two in between days were used for aerobic type exercise days which included walking or running. No suggested weight activity was done those days. Two days off were allowed each week. Walking or running was very difficult for me under Walt's program and I could not understand why. I thought I was a perfectly healthy human being at that stage with no major or minor illness in sight.

Walt carefully began with me on his best days in between practice with his team's daily athlete injury sessions and doctor calls. The sessions were always three days per week. The established days began as Monday, Wednesday and Friday nights.

These days I had latitude if Walt had team duties or if I had client duties. I made a commitment to myself to never let client duties interfere with my workout program. It never did for the full six months of the program.

Walt was floored to the point that he used me as a whipping post for some of the student athletes who regularly missed rehab sessions with him. He would always say to them that I was more committed to getting better than they were. After three weeks of sessions I understood his point. As I became a regular I learned many of the student athletes and coaches names at both institutions Walt worked between.

After vigorously working out with Walt for well over six months Walt told me to join any local fitness center and continue the various exercise programs he had worked with me on. I did just that but visited Walt every three to six months for reinforcement and reassurance just like a doctor. Walt never turned me away. About the time Walt dismissed me one of my closest friends introduced me to a local YMCA. I immediately joined and found that the machines the YMCA maintained were upgraded versions and some the same that Walt had worked with me on.

It became very easy for me to adapt to exercises as new equipment was changed out. As I traveled and look for alternative gyms in case of holiday closures, I found the same to be true using that equipment at other places, that is, it was always an easy transition for me to use other equipment.

This program caused significant improvement in my overall strength. mobility and walking ability. It became a requirement, not an option as my friends and mate repeatedly encouraged me. This created an addiction and love for more workout techniques. I changed to using more machines targeted at my leg muscles first on leg machines such as the treadmill and leg press. This helped immensely and improved my balance. I never let go of any parts of the total program Walt trained and taught me. The steps he built for me at both MBC and Tech always helped with my balance. The YMCA had plastic steps like the ones TV personalities used for workout and dance routines. I was able to buy some from the YMCA and used these additionally at home. This increased mobility a lot and gave me a crutch to use when I needed it.

The local YMCA constantly changed out equipment for more up to date equipment. It always kept updated versions of the more popular machines and brought in more versions that improved your total health. I never found myself unable to use any of the equipment I chose. Instead many members, new and existing were asking me how to use various machines. This always felt good but I knew how I wound up going to the Y and how and why I started exercising regularly after all these years of being idle.

It was nearly two full years before I was diagnosed with m.s after I had begun exercising regularly. The limp remained with me despite vigorous exercising minimum three days per week.

The limp got worse at times when I would neglect exercising every other day as planned. There was still no pain, just the limp which was noticeable to onlookers. Most of the time I did not even know I had a limp. After nursing my limp in this manner for approximately one and one half years, tingling in my legs and some numbness in my feet occurred. This caused me to discuss more in depth with my internist who referred me to a neurologist.

My first neurologist did extensive testing including an mri. He ruled out lime disease, lupus, and treated me with aspirin for six months because the symptoms appeared like a stroke and legions on my brain appeared in the mri. Finally after three months of treatment the first neurologist told me he had ruled out everything except m.s. Therefore, he recommended drug therapy immediately. I did not concede to do this until I obtained a second opinion from a second neurologist. This neurologist took the test and films from the first neurologist and upheld the opinion I had m.s. He recommended immediate drug therapy.

The neurologist placed me on a major drug which required me injecting myself with a needle once per week. I maintained this treatment myself for two years. No other crippling or disabling symptoms occurred during my pre-treatment years nor during the treatment. The neurologist told me to keep exercising. I did without any outside encouragement. I told Walt about the diagnosis and he told me to come by anytime I needed him.

The shots were never easy for me to do myself but I learned to adapt to the process. A nurse was sent all the way from California by my drug company and taught me using oranges. The process was more difficult for my mate than me. She would almost pass out watching me inject myself. As time passed on we both learned it was a "requirement and not an option", a phrase she coined with my drug therapy and exercise routines. My mate and I notice the drugs had short term effects only each week when it came to strength. It did help with the discomfort of tingling and numbness.

My walking grew worse at times and I feared not being able to walk so bad that I delegated job projects to couriers or even sent for lunch at the fun times I used to crave to come around each day. Despite the walking problems I never gave up on exercising. The routines Walt gave me and the new routines I learned through trials helped greatly but I did not make the time to do them daily. After going on in this manner for nearly two years, my faith in God showed me a more comprehensive way. I chose a natural approach that kept me exercising more often and it showed immediate signs of improvement including walking mobility and strength.

This carefully chosen approach was not done all at once. I was so cautious and careful I scared myself often. I would not do anything without first praying sometimes many times a day. Secondly I read and re-read everything I tried. I always sought re-enforcement reading and medical journals as often as I could daily. This became a part-time job and hobby. It was not at all boring nor laborious. Instead I always sensed a call to duty.

Walt's systematic weight resistance training program was always maintained as my weekly foundation exercise program. However, I learned to adjust frequencies of repetitions and used other equipment that targeted areas of my body that certain machines appeared to have helped stimulate my muscles and body parts better. These included machines aimed at resistance, leg press type machines. This coincided with Walt's treatment that he called manual resistance which required him using his body against my legs. This worked and caused me to think and rethink about researching m.s., its causes and cures. Even though medical experts had told me it was no cure, it did not discourage me from seeking means to get better.

For nearly five years after working with Walt I found myself never giving in to health discomforts, personal interferences nor schedule conflicts, whether job or personal. My clients always rallied around me with my schedule even though they had no idea what I was doing with my life. I got many compliments during these years from clients about my improved physique. Everyone wanted to know how I maintained.

Applying the same type of start to finish exercise routines on the circuit training it continued to make me feel and look better. My arms included free weights with curls, dominating legs included leg lifts and I later added two abdominal machines and bike routines which extended over ten minutes alone. A floor exercise routine, which simulated the Olympic style benches, palates was created and used by me. Pilates was not even in my vocabulary at the time.

Next I always applied leg press exercises, arm rowing, and curls. Walt and research taught me to begin with stretches each session and end with warm down equipment. My warm down equipment was usually my steps or bike. Tingling and discomfort disappeared and total body strength and toning improved noticeably.

Walt's coaching and teaching had led me to do a run/walk on my in between exercise days. It occurred to me that walking was regarded as an aerobic activity by many of the medical journals and gyms I attended. Co-workers encouraged me to try walking. Daily trials of walking began for three consecutive months. This appeared to begin doing something miraculous to me. It made me feel like wanting to walk everyday and as often as I could.

The first problem with walking was choosing a suitable place. Many things were tried to find the right spot including going back to my old secluded neighborhood track. It didn't feel comfortable because there were people around noticing me as I limped around the track. Another familiar track near my workplace was tried but this didn't fit because older and more people attended this track and noticed me even more. This was too uncomfortable. The problem was distraction not ashamed of myself. Everybody wanted to talk and ask why you were limping. Shying away from medical discussions which detracted from what I set out to do became my trademark. As I continued to do this I found out it was one of the best strategies I could have employed. Oh yes, it sure avoided a lot of arguments.

A bell went off in my head one morning after nearly a week of trying to find a suitable place to walk. As I left for work I chose to look at my odometer and the distance it took me to go around our parking lot. Little did I know this was a perfectly, paved circle that extended one half mile around. Also there was more paved area adjacent to this spot if I chose it. It was almost perfect and private. Also, it was a gated community for safety.

Rain and cold did not stop me from walking. Yes, even ridiculously cold mornings did not stop me from my mission. Dressing properly for weather conditions rose to the top of my to-do list. This led me to buy more, suitable gear including gloves and toll caps. Young ladies in the gym asked me, you walked even when it got cold? Reluctantly, I told them yes.

My walking not only improved but the length of time I could walk and the distance was no longer a problem. My walking pace was not fast as I wanted to but I was so happy I could walk again without a cane or any time of help aid. My balance improved noticeably and people along the streets stopped looking at me like I was the neighborhood drunk. You see, multiple sclerosis severely affects your balance. People stopped talking talk about my limp as much as they used to. These were signs to me I was improved by exercising. M.S. had placed me on a mission and I never forgot that.

Even though strength training exercises that Walt had taught me and limited walking had shown me huge improvements in my overall mobility, balance and walking, I felt like more could be done. Considering my achievements, I continued researching further techniques that affect the muscles and walking. Gary Walker's work and books became of interest to me during my search for more knowledge on walking and its impacts on bettering my quality of life. He was regarded as the foremost authority on walking. Mr. Yanker and Kathy Burton teamed with a group of 50 doctors and health professionals to present their findings in a series of seven books called "Walking Medicine."

In one of Mr. Walker's books he described walking as "the best natural remedy for a broad spectrum of illnesses, from life-threatening disorders like heart disease and diabetes, to chronic conditions like arthritis and depression. Even everyday problems like stress, lack of energy, and weight gain showed positive results from walking. He further stated "that no food, medicine nor vitamin can provide the same steady healing power." The word "steady" stood out immediately to me. My formal education and work background required that I remained steady, consistent and balanced in my approaches to work. Therefore, this made sense to me in furthering my approaches to get better.

The authors also stated that the "prime advantage of walking is its sheer simplicity. Other exercise programs fail because they cause overexertion and high-impact injuries, or because they require expensive equipment and special venues." Exercise walking as Mr. Yanker appropriately called his work "is not only easy, safe, and inexpensive, but can be done in any locale."

The authors' chart on how walking helps the body systems was particularly interesting to me. This chart is depicted on the next page of his book. I immediately saw noticeable benefits in certain areas listed in the chart. These included the central nervous system, flexibility, reduction in stiffness of joints, improvement in balance and increased energy.

In one of their Walking Medicine books, the authors stated that "walking is probably the best health remedy for adding more and better years to your life." They equate the benefits of walking as significant as quitting smoking or reducing cholesterol. Also they cited walking as a contributor in reducing the need for medications in fighting problems associated with arthritis, diabetes, and high blood pressure. Naturally, most interesting to me was the authors featured statements on multiple sclerosis. They stated that m.s. responds to many of the same exercise and walking solutions as does arthritis, although it is not an arthritic disease. My findings in my own research supported their interesting but limited section on the topic of multiple sclerosis.

The authors' statements about exercising too strenuously during warm weather had already been experienced by me. In fact, this had happened on two occasions during warm weather. Eventually these were known to me as multiple sclerosis related problems. My first encounter was prior to my diagnosis as an m.s. patient. The setting was a trip in a hot southern city where temperatures reached 98 degrees. My friend and I had walked several blocks in these temperatures when I felt faint. Also it became difficult for me to maintain my balance while walking. I grew more clumsy with each step and repeatedly stumbled. The second incident occurred years later in Atlanta during temperatures of 95 degrees plus at a PGA golf tournament. The same friend was with me and saw the symptoms coming on. Help was immediately called and the service providers of the tournament carried me back to the clubhouse.

Neither occurrence was known to me as multiple sclerosis related incidents at the time of each. No medical treatment was sought for either incidence. However, my friend repeatedly chastised me to seek further medical treatment for incidence one. After I got home, I did for incidence one which later led to a series of tests and my eventual diagnosis as an m.s. patient. Later, I read about exacerbations and the doctor's explanations for such occurrences or multiple sclerosis attacks. I knew that was what occurred.

A chart of various exercises Walt gave me and trained me to do is located at the end of this section. It is strongly recommended that you use a certified trainer to show you how to do these and give you the frequency before trying any of them.

JOSEPH L. WILSON IS NOT A PHYSICIAN AND DOES NOT CLAIM TO ACT AS ONE. IT IS RECOMMENDED THAT ANY READER SUFFERING FROM ANY MEDICAL CONDITION CONSULT HIS OR HER PHYSICIAN.

WORKOUT A		
Bench press		
Squat		
Cable row		
Leg extension		
Military press		
Bent-knee incline situp		
Biceps curl		
Standing calf raise		

WORKOUT B		
Lat pulldown		
Lying leg curl		
Dip		
Leg press		
Lateral raise		
Back extension		
Dumbbell shrug		
Reverse crunch		

2

WHAT ARE THE RIGHT THINGS TO EAT AND DRINK

NUTRITION-FOOD

My nutritional habits were totally overhauled. I had to make a choice either to get well, live longer or die crippled and mangled up slowly. These choices were compared to that of a soldier at war. Each day I had to be totally aware of my surroundings or face unwanted uncertainty. Nutritionally, this meant changing all my food and drinking habits. Yes, all, water, sodas, alcoholic beverage contents and juice. The alternative appeared pretty obvious to me.

I could have gotten worse instead of better if I did nothing or if I didn't follow a logical plan to its conclusion. The area of nutrition appeared foreign to me. Extensive research was required on my part. In my research material I always sought the resources of highly authoritative and proven experts in their fields.

Some prior reading on my part about "miracle cures" and foods you can find in the bible prepared me for some future moves. I took off on massive research with my limited knowledge of diet habits and what it would take to eat and drink right. Eating right kept me from getting ill and avoided side effects in doing so. One of my favorite biblical faith stories contained some insight. This insight came from listening to one of my favorite ministers of the gospel challenge the congregation to read the background chapters of Daniel.

It was Daniel, chapter 1, verses 8 through 15. In these verses, "Daniel asked the guard appointed by the chief official of Nebuchadnezzar not to serve the food and drink assigned by the king. Instead Daniel requested vegetables to eat and water to drink for ten days. At the end of ten days Daniel and his three friends looked healthier and better than any of the young men who ate the king's royal food." If you continue in this book of Daniel you read the familiar story of Christ's deliverance of these three men, Shadrach, Meshach and Abednego from the king's fiery furnace.

In my daily quest for knowledge I heard about vegetarian dieting. Vegetables and fruit were childhood and adulthood favorites of mine so the transition appeared easy. Leaving out dairy products, I began experimenting at breakfast time and replaced the dairy products with oatmeal and fruit. Fruit consisted of grapes and bananas on a daily basis. Lunch had become mostly vegetable plates with at least one green leafy vegetable per day. Most of the times this leafy vegetable was my favorite, collard greens.

Why a green leafy vegetable? My internist had previously asked me if I had someone who could cook me a green leafy vegetable each day. He told me if I did this with regularity I would see huge changes in the digestion of my food and avoid problems such as constipation and hemorrhoids. I remembered when I heeded his advice, good results happened.

Walt had called my exercise program a rehab program. Piggybacking off Walt's successful portion of my total program I called my trial period with my nutritional changes an extended rehab period. During my extended rehab period I even started cooking vegetables for lunch myself. Most of the times it wasn't too tasty but I knew I had to keep trying. Each time I tried I got better and better. The food began to taste good.

Thanks to Dr. Rho for her recipes in her book such as her barbecued salmon for health taste tricks. Instead of Dr. Rho's juices and no barbeque sauce, I added my own juices picked from the favorites I had begun experimenting with as part of my juicing program. My favorite had become apple-carrot juice. My office staff even tried my barbecued salmon and liked it. No paramedics were needed and this began as a regular once per week deal at lunch in the office. One young lady from Louisiana took her own version of my recipe home. I knew she could cook having come from Louisiana. Improvising was a cinch for her. Furthermore, she was my band of courage to keep on trying to cook and get better at it.

Dinner became my most challenging meal because it was difficult for me to accept the research that I should eat less for dinner than at lunch. Since childhood I always had been taught that you ate your biggest meal of the day at dinner and ate a light lunch. Oftentimes during my trials dinner was a subway vegetarian sub or tuna sub, never any other type of meat entree. Potato chips, or a self prepared baked potato or my own prepared salad were added as the sides. Other times it was a fruit medley for dinner. This manner was easily accepted because it required less cooking and preparation of me. My mean, as in good salad and fruit medley were really tasty.

Eating in the above manner became a normal way of life after about three months. No foods were microwaved when I cooked. As close to 100% natural and wholesome foods as I could locate by reading all labels before purchasing became the norm. Even the meaning and nutritional aspect of organic food purchases came into my shopping for food. The places I chose to eat out became as scarce as my could eat food list. Basically, my food intake became fruits, vegetables and grains of all kinds. Fish products remained on my diet except shellfish which I rarely cared for any way except shrimp. Shrimp remained my weakness and I continued eating about once every two weeks with caution and guilt.

One thing became certain to me after a lot of trials and experimentation with different foods. Three meals per day excluding snacks were a must. This was a tough assignment for me because I rarely ate three meals per day when somebody else cooked for me over twenty years since my childhood. This became a huge challenge for me anyway because it became very noticeable to me and other acquaintances that weight loss occurred when I didn't maintain three full meals per day.

Snacking was never the problem. Rarely did I snack as a child or during my collegiate years. People close to me who saw my diet habits encouraged me to try snacking. Added to my must eat list at snacks were peanuts, almonds, potato chips, pecans and peanut butter crackers. Fruits were added at times. All of the items I tried were cholesterol free items and nutritionally sound according to most medical experts.

Chicken was another hard area to leave alone. During my life of forty plus years eating chicken from either the family poultry yard or from the neighborhood grocery market was a must. Chicken was extremely healthy I was always told and must be included in your diet. However, I lost my taste for chicken while experimenting with salads during my rehab period. No other meats were even thought as replacements during my experimental eating habits. Salt and pepper were used sparingly. No other spices were used except mustard and mayonnaise on subs.

During my close to vegetarian nutritional habits, I left all other meats alone except some fish. Why fish? Early in my reading, I discovered that some studies had been done and showed people who ate lots of fish products had shown less signs of m.s. arthritic conditions than people who did not eat much fish products in their diets. Further, some of my reading material recommended fish products as a natural help with m.s. conditions. This was accepted by me with no medical assistance or advice.

Strategic at planning my lunch and dinner meals I included a lot of fish products for the entire extended rehab period, a two year period. When I did not include fish at lunch, I ate an entire vegctable plate. On most days that I ate a vegetable plate lunch, I included fish products at dinner. Most of the times I cooked the fish.

This was the biggest risk I took in my diet, consuming fish products. Some of the leading experts I researched during my extended rehab period said no meat products. There were all sorts of reasons not to eat fish nor any other meat products. No one countered what I had heard or read about m.s. and fish. Dr. Joel Fuhrman's "Eat to Live" book said that "the bottom line, choose fish over animal products, but be aware that the place where it was caught, and the type of fish matters. Never eat high-mercury content fish because it has been shown to increase heart attack risk." Dr. Fuhrman even placed a chart in his book apparently from the FDA that showed fish with the highest and lowest mercury Levels. This chart showed tuna in the high mercury category. Needless to say this chart changed my fish diet habits. However, it was comforting to know that there were other fish on the chart I was regularly eating in the low mercury level. These included salmon, my favorite, tilapia and trout.

No pork, beef products, nor dairy products were eaten during my extended rehab period. Again, this was not a hard choice for me except at breakfast time.

Searching for a way to turn away from grits, bacon, sausage, egg and cheese was an enormous undertaking. These had been a part of my diet since childhood. After leaving my home-town, I got ridiculous consuming big amounts of each. However, I began my approach at breakfast primarily with oatmeal and fruits daily. Grapes and bananas were daily choices. Apples, strawberries and peaches were other favorites. Occasionally, I topped off oatmeal with honey or raisins. This gave it some taste and remained nutritious.

Desserts were absent from my meals the entire extended rehab period, twenty four months. There were no more of my favor-ites-peach cobbler, pound cake, chocolate cake, apple pie, sweet potato pie nor pineapple cake. After at least two of my female gym partners told me they had successfully stopped eating desserts over two years previously without health challenges, I proceeded without caution.

All of my reading showed sugar did nothing to help me. Dr. Day's book, "Getting Started On Getting Well", stated that sugar and sugar substitutes suppressed the immune system for hours and robbed the body of vitamins and minerals. They promoted cancer growth.

Limited knowledge of diabetes caused more curiosity about sugar. It was known as sugar diabetes in my neighborhood as a youngster growing up. One of my great aunts, my grandmother's sister, developed this bad disease. This was one of my favorite aunts whom I spent I great deal of time around growing up. This aunt gave me special carpentry job assignments around her home primarily during summer months and paid me. She made sure I spent the money wisely on clothes each week even if it was only an accessory. Having watched her suffer during my childhood became my biggest motive for no sugar in my diet.

In my meals I prepared myself I added natural ingredients with nutritional research. Some of these were parsley, garlic, rosemary, thyme and onions. Garlic and onions were not a part of my diet habits nor meals for forty plus years. The smell of both discredited them for me eating them. However, research showed me these were must items for a variety of health reasons. Included in these reasons were improved arthritic and multiple sclerosis symptoms.

Nutrition-Juicing

The idea of juicing came from reading several leading medical and fitness publications in doctors' offices and the gym I frequented. This addition of juice made everything make sense to me. It appeared that the food did its part to keep you energized and certain parts of your body working properly. Juice appeared as the gas and oil parts (similar to an automobile) to do its part to keep things lubricated and running. Research showed me the juices got rid of toxins daily. The labels of the juices I used told me that the juices contained antioxidants. Later I learned that this was an excellent means of removing poisonous substances from my body on a daily basis.

My initial concerns were how much juice and which kinds. Initially I peaked out at eight (8) ounce glasses of juice per day for three months. Remember I also had to drink water. That seemed like a lot and it was. However, research showed me this was a must to begin in this manner. I had no medical supervision nor case studies nearby to lean on. The spirit of God continued to lead me and let me know in all of my reading this was the right approach. Dr. Lorraine day's work inspired me the most of all my reading because of her Christ like approach.

Carefully I chose which kinds of juice according to what I liked and the type of label contents of each. I knew carrot juice was going to be a part of whatever I did because of its cancer fighting credentials Dr. Day gave it. Deviation from Dr. Day's recommendation to do your own juicing was necessary for me because I had to maintain my work habits while doing this. Therefore, I chose to purchase my juices. After nearly one month of research I found the answer, freshly prepared juices at nearby local grocers brought in every day.

Reliance on labels showed me the freshness of products and its contents. The internet assisted me in telling me of the credibility of the companies and the purpose of each juice. Persistence led me to one company that was eighty (80) plus years old and boasted in its advertising as a four generation company. Common sense told me this had cured and kept a lot of people functioning for a long time. This product became my hub for juices.

All labels contained clear indications the juices I used were always 100% juice, not made from concentrate. Additional juice types were carefully chosen with my likes and dislikes but primarily with the function of the juice. Apple-carrot, green vegetable-fruit juices, varieties of smoothies, tomato and orange juices were among my favorites. It is worth noting that my juices were carefully chosen by their contents. Those ingredients were always researched to determine what health areas of the body the ingredients targeted to make better. Rapidly my zeal for knowledge expanded to such things as wheat grass, spinach, spirulina and other contents. Some of these things I had never heard of prior to researching.

Dr. Day's tips on digestion worked for me. Drinking occurred minimum thirty (30) minutes before eating anything and minimum one hour before I drink again. It occurred to me this was a way to properly allow nutrients to digest and do what they were intended to do.

The use of juice immediately showed me positive body effects and health improvements. This is where I began to look at diagrams of the digestive system and its functions. Later in this section of nutrition I have placed a pre approved diagram of the digestive system and how it works. Reproduction of this section was encouraged by the National Digestive Diseases Clearinghouse, a service of the National Institute of Diabetes and Digestive and Kidney Diseases (NIDDK).

Juicing appeared to have improved every area of my body's natural functions. Notes were compared with my internist, urologist and neurologist. All encouraged me to keep doing what I was doing and don't make any changes.

Every since early adulthood I had been faced with an unpleasant case of mild constipation. It would always come and go. When I sought medical treatment as a young adult it was always dismissed as hemorrhoids. The medical experts always reacted as it was a condition that everyone was going to have at least once in their lives. Therefore, I always accepted and dismissed this condition as something normal.

After reaching forty plus, medical experts decided I better have a colonostrophy. This was done around 2001 and the specialist doctor who performed the procedures again dismissed the only condition he discovered as just hemorrhoids. Again I did nor said nothing different as the doctor did. It did not even occur to me until researching my m.s. medical condition I should have asked the doctor questions like what caused hemorrhoids or will hemorrhoids lead into something more serious. Instead I was always relieved to hear the medical experts sigh with relief and dismiss the condition as only hemorrhoids.

While researching my m. s. condition it occurred to me that my hemorrhoid state was more serious than I thought. This occurred in parts of the digestive system. Everything in the digestive system had to work in order for me to do the things necessary to get better, eating right, juicing, and consuming water. These things had to be properly eliminated. My little knowledge of how often or when quickly was replaced through actual trials and reading more. Some knowledgeable women who heard me talk about eating and drinking more healthy food and drink things told me to look at young babies. These young women said that every time you feed them they have a bowel movement. They all used the phrase, typical man; he never noticed his own kids because he didn't have to participate in the cleanup stage that much.

I got the message, however, and realized that whatever I put in my body was going to come out. Therefore, I turned my research to the type of experts who I relied on the most during my rehab period. At the top of my list was Dr. Lorraine Day. Dr. Day's material gave me digestive tips that didn't mean as much medically as it would have to a medical expert. But I accepted her approach to her problem. That is, I drank no less than one hour after a meal and ate no less than thirty minutes after drinking. Again, I didn't understand all the whys medically but I knew it had a lot to do with digestion. Dr. Day's book "Getting Started On GettingWell" talked about constipation in a serious light, cancer causing condition. My condition was not known to cause cancer but cancer was one of the diseases I feared. Having already been diagnosed with m.s. meant to me I could possibly catch one more major disease that could be devastating. Needless to say, I had all the incentive I needed to continue with research and good habits to avoid cancer, heart conditions, diabetes, kidney problems and everything else imaginable.

Huge research was done by me on the digestive system and as a result I felt like the next few pages inserted into this book should be made available for reading to everyone interested in getting well from a degenerative condition. Remember, this condition medical experts termed as a noninfectious disease. A degenerative disease according to medical experts has its origin from deficiencies and problems stirred up inside the body. This definition gave me a ray of hope. It meant to me that I could be cured of my disease even if medical experts said there was no known cure. Ultimately it meant to me I had to stay committed to God above and follow the chosen course to conclusion.

Both infectious and degenerative diseases have as their origin an outside source, whether bacteria, viruses, yeasts, fungi, or other pathogenic organisms (infectious diseases) or toxic substances and acids (degenerative diseases). More in depth reading is recommended medically by me on these subjects to get a better grasp. An interesting internet quote was posted by a medical group, "If doctors of today do not become the nutritionists of tomorrow, then the nutritionists of today will become the doctors of tomorrow". The Rockefeller institute of medical research is credited.

At the plateau of my nutritional successes, I ran across the nutritional work and accomplishments of Dr. Stuart Berger, M.D. Dr. Berger's work had been documented in his own series of books, How To Be Your Own Nutritionist, Immune Power Diet, the Southampton Diet and other work. Scanning some of Dr. Berger's work reassured me that what I accomplished should be documented and presented to others for their reading digestion.

In Dr. Berger's "How To Be Your Own Nutritionist", I took particular interest in his comments that "you know your body better than anyone else possibly could". This premise was one of the building blocks of my thinking all along in my approach and search for knowledge. Dr. Berger offered several other interesting comments in this same book including "the right foods protect you as nature intended them to while others sabotage your finely balanced system." An interesting section entitled "nutrients and your body's systems" appeared near the end of Dr. Berger's book. This section gave me a diagram for each of the body's major health systems. Each of his diagrams includes various help nutrients to get better if properly used. These diagrams supported much of the research I had previously done to get better and echoed many of the types of nutrients I utilized.

Dr. Berger's work clarified much of my own thinking about the approach I had taken through various reports and studies. This immediately introduced a positive new challenge for me and steered me on a course for more research and personal experimentation.

Now, let me clarify what I meant by my own thinking in my approach to get better. No, I did not have any aspiration to ever be a medical doctor nor was it my intent to cure myself. Tidbits of information I obtained from various doctors and radio talk show hosts on medical shows gave me the incentive and knowledge to do my part to help my doctor. This meant for me to do everything the medical society and other reliable resources said do to obtain optimum health for myself before the need to see a doctor.

Whoever wanted side effects? After all, I never heard of good side effects. My approach always sought out the side effects that might occur with whatever I decided to eat or drink. Further, I accepted no one's advice or reading topic without researching further myself to ensure it made good common sense. Experimentation was never attempted. However, if an approach on something I tried appeared to not work as well as I thought, I changed. On the other hand, there were times some things appeared to work better. So, I changed and tried it a different way.

An example was my intake of fish products. My approach became a weekly habit and most of time during my extended rehab period it was two to three times per week I ate fish, mostly salmon. Also, an example can be made of my fluid intake. Desperately, I tried to always to drink eight regular eight ounce glasses of water per day and eight to 11 glasses of 100 % juice per day. These standards had been spelled out by me for myself as the standards of excellence to achieve positive results to what I was attempting. Some days I succeeded but most days I did not make it. Therefore, I became very comfortable and proud of myself by making it to consume 7 and one half glasses of water per day and eight glasses of 100% juice per day during my extended rehab period.

Around the time I found Dr. Stuart Berger's work, I discovered the written work of Gladys Lindbergh and her daughter, Judy Lindbergh McFarland. Both Dr. Berger's and nutritionist Lindbergh's work were used to support what had already happened to my health. Their works reassured me that better nutritional habits played a vital role in helping me to live a better quality of life.

Gladys Lindbergh was a leading nutritionist who founded the Lindbergh Nutrition Center. Her daughter was so in awe of her work to find answers for her family health concerns which led to bigger and better things for people of all walks of life, she co-authored the book "Take Charge Of Your Health". This amazing story of her mother's pioneering efforts in nutrition is not only intriguing but inspiring to all who have experienced illness over an extended time. Also, it remains an invaluable lesson to all non believers in helping your doctors find cures for you and your family.

Her daughter admirably described her mother as the "wheat germ lady" in chapter one of this book. Chapter two is another one of the premises that launched my search for knowledge about my own health and how I could live a better quality of life. I'm referring to "what did our ancestors do different from us?"

The term degenerative disease was first brought to my attention by Dr. Lorraine Day's work. This topic was dealt with in chapter three of "Take Charge Of Your Health". It is stated in the book that degenerative diseases are not caused by viruses, bacteria or parasites. The real killer is malnutrition-more commonly referred to as diabetes, cancer, arthritis, etc. These diseases are usually caused by the absence of some substance (vitamin, mineral or trace element) cited by medical doctors, nutritionist Lindbergh referenced in her own research. Dr.

Day's work introduced me to the idea that my disease, multiple sclerosis fit the degenerative disease category.

This meant to me I could be cured if I really committed myself to getting well.

Particularly, I liked the section in nutritionist Lindbergh's book on the immune system, chapter 9. It is stated in the book that malnutrition leads to a weakening or suppression of the immune system. She termed it as "any disorder of nutrition". This chapter led me to a word my grandparents often used as I grew up, resistance. They would say when I caught colds, or fever, that boy's resistance is low. By the way, I was rarely sick as a child. My entire childhood was spent with my grandparents, my father's parents. Usually, my grandparents applied some old fashioned remedy or only took me to the medical doctor when their remedies did not show them immediate signs of improvement.

My grandmother, Essie Mae and grandfather Dave, reared me from birth in a small rural town near Albany, Georgia, Dawson, Georgia. Grandmother Essie Mae, whom I affectionately called "mama", instilled in me and all neighborhood children many principles to live by. These principles left no room for negotiation. My cousins and I called these principles, Essiemae's do's and don'ts. Her most notable food (nutritional) principle was never substitute junk food as a meal. Junk food to her meant candy, cookies, sandwiches, chips and sodas. A meal meant vegetables, bread cooked from scratch and meat cooked on a stove top. Dessert (something sweet) was rare, maybe once every two weeks.

Both of my grandparents lived in excess of 70 years old and I was around both of them until death. Their deaths appeared to be very young in age numerically to me and nearby residents. Most of the residents I grew up around in that community lived to be in excess of 80 to 90 years old. One of my aunts that was my favorite Sunday dinner partner when I didn't eat at home lived to be 97 years old.

Apparently, the immune system did just what Dr. Berger and nutritionist Lindbergh all implied. In my words, you keep it well maintained, it will keep you well. This sounded like the jingle used by auto mechanics, maintain your oil changes regularly and this will take care of your engine for years to come.

Menus-Extended Rehab Period

When I shared with friends, associates, gym partners and some other acquaintancies I had begun writing a book about health habits, it was suggested to me more than once to include menus on how I ate. In my own mind, this was already included in the nutritional section of the book. After wrestling with myself, I decided it would be more beneficial to highlight this in a better format. Following are some of my nutritional habits during my extended rehab period.

Breafast List

Strawberries
Large bowl grapes
One whole banana
Sliced apples
Sliced cantaloupe during season
1 Peach during season
Large bowl oatmeal
A smoothie (Breakfast meal by itself)
100 % whole wheat toast

A combination of most of the above fruits were eaten every breakfast. Grapes and oatmeal were rarely absent from a breakfast meal. A smoothie was substituted as a meal rarely one day of the week that I chose not to cook oatmeal. I even felt guilty that I was depriving my system of something when I did this with a smoothie alone even though most of my research material said this was okay.

Lunch

Vegetarian plate consisting of any combination of the following vegetables-

Collards
Turnips
Corn boiled on the cob or cream style
Green beans
Lima beans

Carrot soufflé
Yams
Sliced tomatoes
Occasional okra with tomato and corn mixed
Broccoli
Carrots
Peas green or black eyed
Baked potato

Added to any of the above vegetables certain days that I didn't eat a vegaetarian plate
Were grilled salmon two to three days per week
Or grilled talapia once per week
Or rice or baked potato

Lunch was a struggle initially because I was not accustomed to eating a large lunch. I used to skip lunch a lot when I worked in the corporate world. Weight fluctuation after being diagnosed with m.s. stopped the missing lunches because I was placed on medication. My mate soon convinced me to eat to maintain my weight.

Dinner

Fruit medley (once per every two weeks)
Tuna submarine sandwich
Grilled salmon
Baked potato
Boiled corn on the cob
Potato chips (baked)

Broccoli (steamed)
Carrots (steamed)
Rice (brown)
Sliced tomato
Vegetable garden salad, usually spinach or lettuce with tomatoes and heath food selected salad dressing

I stuck mainly with vegetables only 80% of the time. Occasionally I added fish items for dinner. I never ate meat items (fish) for both lunch and dinner on the same day. That became a practicing habit.

Daily liquid intake

My liquid intake became just as important to me as my meals. Never had I considered drinking was so important before I began researching my medical condition. No other liquids were consumed by me during the extended rehab period except 100% juices and water.

Early a.m. one glass of water
Following the water no less than thirty minutes, one glass of 100% orange juice.

Breakfast
No less than one hour after breakfast, one glass of either 100% carrot juice or 100% apple-carrot juice.
No less than thirty minutes after last juice 1 glass of green leafy vegetable juice with barley.

Lunch

One hour after lunch, more juice usually 100% tomato juice or carrot juice.

For next few hours after waiting thirty minutes apart I continued juicing and some water mixed in between. Juices were 100% carrot, apple-carrot or green leafy vegetable juice with barley included.

Dinner

One glass of water no less than one hour after dinner

And one glass 100% apple-carrot juice for night cap minimum thirty minutes after water.

NUTRITION-WATER

Water is so natural that it had always been taken for granted by me. It was normal growing up that I knew to go get a glass of water when I got thirsty. Quenching my thirst was always the reason I wanted water. Never had the idea of drinking water because it was healthy for you enter my mine before I began my research to get better from m.s. conditions. Everywhere I turned, books, periodicals in doctor offices, newspaper articles, television, and radio indicated it was healthy to drink water and plenty of it each day.

It occurred to me in the early ninetics to get a water fountain for home and my office. This appeared to be the faddish thing to do. Again, health was not my primary aim. However, my family and I had become a ware that water pipes in your residence and office may not be safe to drink from because of many reasons. This was a major concern. During my health search so many indicators and facts appeared to me until I felt like cave man. My knowledge and respect for water grew each day.

My body responded to water as I tried an approach that fit my daily routine during my extended rehab period. Each day I began early when I got up with one to one and one half glass of water. Every other day was my normal gym day in the early morning. This allowed me to fit in another full glass immediately after leaving the gym. On days I did not go to the gym I always fit in a second glass of water early mornings usually after arriving at the office. After that, I fit water drinking into my liquid intake schedule after lunch. Juice and water were drank one hour after lunch until dinner time. This liquid intake continued every thirty minutes with regularity. After dinner I usually drank no more than one glass of water before bed time. Sometimes if I had not made my goal of minimum 7.5 glasses of water per day, I made efforts to sip some more water during the night but never more than one full glass per night. After all, I really looked forward to sleeping each night during my post rehab period. Eating and drinking well played its role in helping me to sleep well.

In the beginning drinking more than three glasses of water per day was a real hurdle. It took me about three to four weeks for my body to accept five full glasses of water per day. After reaching this plateau, I began sailing. It was not uncommon for me to take in eight to ten glasses of water per day during a full week.

You could not have paid me to believe before my real life experiences about the role water played in my eliminating process. Sure every one understood the urinary process. However, it was quite intriguing to observe water's full role without anybody telling me a thing. No doctor had even come close to telling me the things I learned and observed. This caused me to go to the library and do some digestive system searching. Diagrams became interesting to me to locate internal organs and study their roles. This clearly made me appreciate their functions and focused my search for food and drink that assisted these body parts to function better naturally. All the research showed water was the sentimental favorite to assist each body part to function properly without man made help aids.

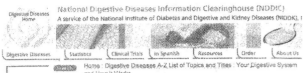

National Digestive Diseases Information Clearinghouse (NDDIC)

A service of the National Institute of Diabetes and Digestive and Kidney Diseases (NIDDK), I

Digestive Diseases | Statistics | Clinical Trials | In Spanish | Resources | Order | About Us

Home : Digestive Diseases A-Z List of Topics and Titles : Your Digestive System and How It Works

Email To A Friend ✉

Print This Page 🖨

Spanish Version

Your Digestive System and How It Works

On this page:

- Why is digestion important?
- How is food digested?
- How is the digestive process controlled?

The digestive system is a series of hollow organs joined in a long, twisting tube from the mouth to the anus (see figure). Inside this tube is a lining called the mucosa. In the mouth, stomach, and small intestine, the mucosa contains tiny glands that produce juices to help digest food.

Two solid organs, the liver and the pancreas, produce digestive juices that reach the intestine through small tubes. In addition, parts of other organ systems (for instance, nerves and blood) play a major role in the digestive system.

[Top]

Why is digestion important?

When we eat such things as bread, meat, and vegetables, they are not in a form that the body can use as nourishment. Our food and drink must be changed into smaller molecules of nutrients before they can be absorbed into the blood and carried to cells throughout the body. Digestion is the process by which food and drink are broken down into their smallest parts so that the body can use them to build and nourish cells and to provide energy.

[Top]

How is food digested?

Digestion involves the mixing of food, its movement through

the digestive tract, and the chemical breakdown of the large molecules of food into smaller molecules. Digestion begins in the mouth, when we chew and swallow, and is completed in the small intestine. The chemical process varies somewhat for different kinds of food.

Movement of Food Through the System

The large, hollow organs of the digestive system contain muscle that enables their walls to move. The movement of organ walls can propel food and liquid and also can mix the contents within each organ. Typical movement of the esophagus, stomach, and intestine is called peristalsis. The action of peristalsis looks like an ocean wave moving through the muscle. The muscle of the organ produces a narrowing and then propels the narrowed portion slowly down the length of the organ. These waves of narrowing push the food and fluid in front of them through each hollow organ.

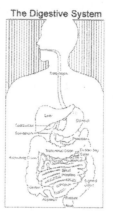

The Digestive System

The first major muscle movement occurs when food or liquid is swallowed. Although we are able to start swallowing by choice, once the swallow begins, it becomes involuntary and proceeds under the control of the nerves.

The esophagus is the organ into which the swallowed food is pushed. It connects the throat above with the stomach below. At the junction of the esophagus and stomach, there is a ringlike valve closing the passage between the two organs. However, as the food approaches the closed ring, the surrounding muscles relax and allow the food to pass.

The food then enters the stomach, which has three mechanical tasks to do. First, the stomach must store the swallowed food and liquid. This requires the muscle of the upper part of the stomach to relax and accept large volumes of swallowed material. The second job is to mix up the food, liquid, and digestive juice produced by the stomach. The lower part of the stomach mixes these materials by its muscle action. The third task of the stomach is to empty its contents slowly into the small intestine.

Several factors affect emptying of the stomach, including the nature of the food (mainly its fat and protein content) and the degree of muscle action of the emptying stomach and the next organ to receive the contents (the small intestine). As the food is digested in the small intestine and dissolved into the juices from the pancreas, liver, and intestine, the contents of the intestine are mixed and pushed forward to allow further digestion.

Finally, all of the digested nutrients are absorbed through the intestinal walls. The waste products of this process include undigested parts of the food, known as fiber, and older cells that have been shed from the mucosa. These materials are propelled into the colon, where they remain, usually for a day or two, until the feces are expelled by a bowel movement.

Production of Digestive Juices

The glands that act first are in the mouth—the salivary glands. Saliva produced by these glands contains an enzyme that begins to digest the starch from food into smaller molecules.

The next set of digestive glands is in the stomach lining. They produce stomach acid and an enzyme that digests protein. One of the unsolved puzzles of the digestive system is why the acid juice of the stomach does not dissolve the tissue of the stomach itself. In most people, the stomach mucosa is able to resist the juice, although food and other tissues of the body cannot.

After the stomach empties the food and juice mixture into the small intestine, the juices of two other digestive organs mix with the food to continue the process of digestion. One of these organs is the pancreas. It produces a juice that contains a wide array of enzymes to break down the carbohydrate, fat, and protein in food. Other enzymes that are active in the process come from glands in the wall of the intestine or even a part of that wall.

The liver produces yet another digestive juice—bile. The bile is stored between meals in the gallbladder. At mealtime, it is squeezed out of the gallbladder into the bile ducts to reach the intestine and mix with the fat in our food. The bile acids dissolve the fat into the watery contents of the intestine, much like detergents that dissolve grease from a frying pan. After the fat is dissolved, it is digested by enzymes from the pancreas and the lining of the intestine.

Absorption and Transport of Nutrients

Digested molecules of food, as well as water and minerals from the diet, are absorbed from the cavity of the upper small intestine. Most absorbed materials cross the mucosa into the blood and are carried off in the bloodstream to other parts of the body for storage or further chemical change. As already noted, this part of the process varies with different types of nutrients.

Carbohydrates. It is recommended that about 55 to 60 percent of total daily calories be from carbohydrates. Some of our most common foods contain mostly carbohydrates. Examples are bread, potatoes, legumes, rice, spaghetti, fruits, and vegetables. Many of these foods contain both starch and fiber.

The digestible carbohydrates are broken into simpler molecules by enzymes in the saliva, in juice produced by the pancreas, and in the lining of the small intestine. Starch is digested in two steps: First, an enzyme in the saliva and pancreatic juice breaks the starch into molecules called maltose; then an enzyme in the lining of the small intestine (maltase) splits the maltose into glucose molecules that can be absorbed into the blood. Glucose is carried through the bloodstream to the liver, where it is stored or used to provide energy for the work of the body.

Table sugar is another carbohydrate that must be digested to be useful. An enzyme in the lining of the small intestine digests table sugar into glucose and fructose, each of which can be absorbed from the intestinal cavity into the blood. Milk contains yet another type of sugar, lactose, which is changed into absorbable molecules by an enzyme called lactase, also found in the intestinal lining.

Protein. Foods such as meat, eggs, and beans consist of giant molecules of protein that must be digested by enzymes before they can be used to build and repair body tissues. An enzyme in the juice of the stomach starts the digestion of swallowed protein. Further digestion of the protein is completed in the small intestine. Here, several enzymes from the pancreatic juice and the lining of the intestine carry out the breakdown of huge protein molecules into small molecules called amino acids. These small molecules can be absorbed from the hollow of the small intestine into the blood and then be carried to all parts of the body to build the walls and other parts of cells.

Fats. Fat molecules are a rich source of energy for the body. The first step in digestion of a fat such as butter is to dissolve it into the watery content of the intestinal cavity. The bile acids produced by the liver act as natural detergents to dissolve fat in water and allow the enzymes to break the large fat molecules into smaller molecules, some of which are fatty acids and cholesterol. The bile acids combine with the fatty acids and cholesterol and help these molecules to move into the cells of the mucosa. In these cells the small molecules are formed back into large molecules, most of which pass into vessels (called lymphatics) near the intestine. These small vessels carry the reformed fat to the veins of the chest, and the blood carries the fat to storage depots in different parts of the body.

Vitamins. Another vital part of our food that is absorbed from the small intestine is the class of chemicals we call vitamins. The two different types of vitamins are classified by the fluid in which they can be dissolved: water-soluble vitamins (all the B vitamins and vitamin C) and fat-soluble vitamins (vitamins A, D, and K).

Water and salt. Most of the material absorbed from the cavity of the small intestine is water in which salt is dissolved. The salt and water come from the food and liquid we swallow and the juices secreted by the many digestive glands.

[Top]

How is the digestive process controlled?

Hormone Regulators

A fascinating feature of the digestive system is that it contains its own regulators. The major hormones that control the functions of the digestive system are produced and released by cells in the mucosa of the stomach and small intestine. These hormones are released into the blood of the digestive tract, travel back to the heart and through the arteries, and return to the digestive system, where they stimulate digestive juices and cause organ movement.

The hormones that control digestion are gastrin, secretin,

and cholecystokinin (CCK):

- **Gastrin** causes the stomach to produce an acid for dissolving and digesting some foods. It is also necessary for the normal growth of the lining of the stomach, small intestine, and colon.

- **Secretin** causes the pancreas to send out a digestive juice that is rich in bicarbonate. It stimulates the stomach to produce pepsin, an enzyme that digests protein, and it also stimulates the liver to produce bile.

- **CCK** causes the pancreas to grow and to produce the enzymes of pancreatic juice, and it causes the gallbladder to empty.

Additional hormones in the digestive system regulate appetite:

- **Ghrelin** is produced in the stomach and upper intestine in the absence of food in the digestive system and stimulates appetite.

- **Peptide YY** is produced in the GI tract in response to a meal in the system and inhibits appetite.

Both of these hormones work on the brain to help regulate the intake of food for energy.

Nerve Regulators

Two types of nerves help to control the action of the digestive system. Extrinsic (outside) nerves come to the digestive organs from the unconscious part of the brain or from the spinal cord. They release a chemical called acetylcholine and another called adrenaline. Acetylcholine causes the muscle of the digestive organs to squeeze with more force and increase the "push" of food and juice through the digestive tract. Acetylcholine also causes the stomach and pancreas to produce more digestive juice. Adrenaline relaxes the muscle of the stomach and intestine and decreases the flow of blood to these organs.

Even more important, though, are the intrinsic (inside) nerves, which make up a very dense network embedded in the walls of the esophagus, stomach, small intestine, and colon. The intrinsic nerves are triggered to act when the walls of the hollow organs are stretched by food. They release many different substances that speed up or delay the movement of food and the production of juices by the digestive organs.

[Top]

National Digestive Diseases Information Clearinghouse

2 Information Way
Bethesda, MD 20892–3570
Email: nddic@info.niddk.nih.gov

The National Digestive Diseases Information Clearinghouse (NDDIC) is a service of the National Institute of Diabetes and Digestive and Kidney Diseases (NIDDK). The NIDDK is part of the National Institutes of Health under the U.S. Department of Health and Human Services. Established in 1980, the Clearinghouse provides information about digestive diseases to people with digestive disorders and to their families, health care professionals, and the public. The NDDIC answers inquiries, develops and distributes publications, and works closely with professional and patient organizations and Government agencies to coordinate resources about digestive diseases.

Publications produced by the Clearinghouse are carefully reviewed by both NIDDK scientists and outside experts.

This publication is not copyrighted. The Clearinghouse encourages users of this publication to duplicate and distribute as many copies as desired.

NIH Publication No. 04–2681
May 2004

[Top]

Digestive Diseases Home | Digestive Diseases A-Z | Statistics | Clinical Trials | In Spanish | Additional Resources | Order Publications | About Us |

Contact Us | NIDDK Health Information

The NDDIC is a service of the National Institute of Diabetes and Digestive and Kidney Diseases, National Institutes of Health

National Digestive Diseases Information Clearinghouse

http://digestive.niddk.nih.gov/ddiseases/pubs/yrdd/   8/13/06

2 Information Way
Bethesda, MD 20892--3570
Phone: 1--800--891--5389
Fax: 703--738--4929
Email: nddic@info.niddk.nih.gov

Privacy | Disclaimer | Accessibility

3

SLEEP

It never occurred to me until my extended rehab period that the lack of or more than enough sleep was a major contributor to health problems. During my post rehab period and after extensive reading and internet research, I decided my patterns of sleep should change. Reading various articles in doctors' offices, and authors' work whom I had pursued for the health related areas scared and confused me.

Determination set in as my mission to find my own comfortable natural sleep cycle. Since childhood I never had a problem of relying on someone or an alarm clock to awaken me. This continued even in my collegiate years as well as my marital years. This was a starting point for me mentally. By this I felt like six and one half hours had always been enough sleep for me to function 100 % each day and rise the next morning without some artificial awakening call.

Anything less than six and one half hours per night of sleep presented a problem for me being able to get up timely the next morning. In addition I struggled through my routine the next day if I got less than six and one half hour sleep the previous night. Things like clumsiness out of the norm, irritability, yawning, and making errors in work or in judgment would set in if I got less than six and one half hour sleep per night.

Therefore, I wasn't about to play around with less than six and one half hours of sleep per night. Deciding how to make it work naturally and fit the rest of my new all natural health lifestyle cycle, continue to be effective and efficient at work was my next mountain to climb. Pushing myself all the way without any assistance from a mate or co-worker, I went to bed much earlier than normal for the first six months of my extended rehab period. Target times to go to bed were set at 9:30 to 10:30 per night. This began to take shape and I always felt better the next day.

Sleep was referred to as my new found friend. Concentration on my work projects improved immediately. Increased energy levels were recognized every early morning. These things sparked some ideas. Since work was not an option for me but required to maintain myself and family, a new work schedule trial that fit some previous successful one time long hour work projects was one answer. An early morning work schedule change was the ultimate answer. My shift began early morning hours after 2:30 a.m. and ended eight to ten hours later. An exercise break consisting of both gym activities and walking outside was taken around 6:00 to 7:30 a.m. most mornings.

This new work schedule gave me several huge advantages such as uninterrupted work flow and more concentration time for work projects. Having recognized these advantages triggered other ideas to move certain work to these times of the morning in my schedule. These things really worked and created a better environment for me to deal with questions and answers for staff members during their peak work periods. Their peak periods became my low periods and we developed excellent teamwork concepts from these experiments. At the same time our work productivity and quality improved.

Sleeping in this manner stabilized over a six month period with little deviation. The later time periods of my extended rehab program were similar. Some adjustments and deviations were needed with times and scheduling. For instance. an entertainment or business event scheduled in the night required some slight shifting of other scheduled activities. These usually presented no problem because I was able to prepare for them in advance. This made me appreciate the life of traveling businessmen and athletes.

The most challenging events that disturbed my flow were things that would come up early mornings. This was mainly because most of my activities, work and play, usually began early mornings. Don't forget I had to get exercise and nutrition in. Flexibility and the will to get everything in kept me on course. Many times this meant changing exercise to p.m slots in the gym. This wasn't a problem because I originally trained in the p.m. and continued working out in this manner for over three years.

Nutritionally speaking, I maintained the cautions of most doctors and my research experts. That is, I tried hard to eat my last meal before 8:00 p.m. most nights. This was most difficult because my routine always shifted in just enough to cause me delay eating that last meal. Earlier was suggested to stop and eat by most experts but this was usually not possible for me because most of the time I was still in rest mode. However, by sticking to this rigorous schedule to eat my last meal earlier, my digestive system improved. Rare incidents of sleeplessness because of eating too late occurred.

The type of foods eaten during my last meal was carefully chosen. It usually included some sort of vegetable, carrots, salad, corn, or potato as a base. Eating in this manner appeared to calm me down for the evening and put my digestive tract on hold. There was very little getting up at nights during my six and one half to eight hours sleep. The juicing and water daily intake usually were the reasons for the two to three times of getting up at night.

Other good natural sleep habit improvements were noticed during my extended rehab period. Among them was the lessening or lack of snoring. My mate and family members noticed my improved snoring habits. It was apparent to me that the stress free practices, exercise, eating the right kinds of food and improved sleep habits had all played roles in helping me to sleep better and feel better each day I awake during my extended rehab period.

During my quest for better sleep habits I was introduced to a new friend, rest. All of my life it never occurred to me that there was a distinct difference in rest and sleep. My changed work schedule allowed me more time for myself personally. Each day I began to stop my work flow automatically around 2:00 p.m. if it had not already stopped. This included questions and answers for the staff. The routine that began shortly after this work stoppage was sitting in the customer lounge and listening to soft music.

Around 4:00 p.m. preparations were made for television watching, law or humor related. This became standard and my staff began to respect the time. After all, they sensed no answers would come out of me during those time periods and I was much easier to get along with at all other times of the day. Most of the times I left television watching and drifted into an evening nap. This nap re-energized me and usually pointed me in the direction to either the gym with a friend, visit with a local business friend or spend quality time with my mate.

Needless to say my daughter was the toughest person to convince this period was really a rest period for me without interruption. Usually she had some hot project that she just had to get an answer from me so she could proceed with whatever she was doing, work related or helping somebody. First she saw my answers as procrastination tactics but later she learned to wait until the rest period was over or try before it began. Oh, how rewarding.

4

STRESS-LESS-NESS

Many things were learned after I was made aware of having multiple sclerosis (M.S.). None of these things overshadowed my grasp for knowledge about stress. During a visit to my main internist in 1999, I made him aware of my left leg having a noticeable limp but no pain associated with it. He and I had regularly engaged in conversations of high blood pressure and the effects of poor prostate conditions. This time it was not one of those regular visits for him to give me a lecture and medication, then I'd be on my way. Instead he checked some vital symptoms including muscle strength testing and exclaimed loudly as we continued talking.

As he completed the tests the conversation that caused him to exclaim loudly was regarding stressful events that had occurred in my life around the time the limp began. His exclamation went something like" I knew it, I knew it." Reluctantly, I asked him what did he mean by I knew it? He stated that he and his colleagues for years had suspected stress was the cause of his suspicions for what he thought I had. Even more curious, I asked him, what do you think I have? He never told me directly during that visit, but immediately referred me to a leading neurologist in the local area. After a year long of tests including an MRI first, this doctor announced his suspicions that I had m.s. He stated "suspicions" because m.s. was known as a sneaky disease that was hard to diagnose. Further he stated that his approach had been to rule out other diseases first including stroke.

This neurologist was not the type of professional that readily shared things with me such as causes. Therefore, this made my curiosity about what was happening to me a mission that I must undertake on my own. Remembering my internist comments, these became my first priority. Looking in the mirror each day I focused on those events that the internist and I communicated about. It occurred to me that things such as strife in a close relationship, constant arguments, regular conflicts, uneasiness around people whom you normally enjoy associating with, and other similar events caused what doctors termed stress.

Exercising had become a part of my daily health plan since discovery of the limp. This is what made me initially seek Walt, my old college trainer who was still in the sports training and health field. It appeared strange to me that this limp would never go away completely even though I had become a consistent exercise artist. Just saying stress played a part in causing me to limp was unheard of, unthinkable and not acceptable initially by me.

So I limped on and off for another three plus years before the real causes of m.s. were accepted by me. Realizing that stress played a significant role, efforts to avoid stress became huge in my life. Exercising had saved me from mass health destruction according to my physicians who regularly had seen me during my pre diagnosis and diagnosis years. Even though my health to these medical professionals never became life threatening, they put me on drug therapy. Learning of the potential side effects of drug therapy caused worry for me, stress again.

Avoiding stress during my post rehab years became as important as exercising and nutrition. Concentrated efforts were made to avoid some of the things that I liked doing but I felt were negatively affecting me. These included watching certain types of programs on television and reading the local newspaper for the big events of the day. These events usually had negative implications. Special efforts were made to never watch news events on television for over six months. Television watching and reading the local newspaper were replaced with watching humorous tapes and DVD's that I began collecting. You know it eventually occurred to me that I really didn't miss the television watching especially the news reporting. Most negative events that occurred in the news circulated to me through people who I regularly saw in the gym, client conversations or family conversations.

Fun events were sought on a regular basis and became part of a lifestyle change for me. These included most of the things that I already loved doing, watching sports events, mostly by television, comedy television watching and DVD, quality spiritual programs on television and DVD's. My walking was hampered initially to the point that fear had set in to try and regularly attend these type of events live. My entire life had been spent enjoying these things live but I found an unforgettable alternative which brought me peace of mind. Against all odds, I continued limping to church but missed some other events discussed earlier.

This erased a lot of stress in my life with little effort. Really, I didn't even know at the time this was positively rehabbing me internally and creating a more positive attitude and disposition daily to outsiders. Speaking of outsiders, I contacted all of my friends before I began my post rehab period. These calls were made to let them know that they had done nothing to harm our friendships but I had a plan to get well which would keep me from regularly seeing them but more importantly would keep me from going with them to the events we had shared so many years. These especially included sporting and musical events. The key became consistent and regular telephone conversations to each of them.

Most of my immediate family members had accepted my condition. Therefore, no telephone calls were needed to them. As my daughter would always say, we were bonded for life, so nothing was going to keep us apart, no matter what. Cautious in my approach I never let my long distance relatives know what was going on. However, regular telephone conversations told them enough. They often said by telephone, you really sound like the old Joseph and would put lots of emphasis in their comments. Things like this were my gauges for my progress.

My family near and far had no knowledge of what I was doing during my post rehab period. They had no knowledge of my activities, that is, whether I was going a little or a lot. Whenever asked I kept the conversations positive It occurred to me there were things that connected to overdoing and underdoing.

Therefore, I always sought a happy medium. Fun and church activities were mainstays daily and weekly. However, if I felt pushed I withdrew from going as much. The biggest obstacle I fought with myself was going to church every Sunday and some weeknight special services. These events always brought calmness over my entire mental state and attitude.

Working habits changed. Again I stopped pushing myself beyond unreasonable daily limits. Instead, organization tactics were changed. Things to do worksheets have always been a part of my work environment. Early a.m. before my staff came in became my mode of operation to compile the daily things to do lists for lesser experienced staff and myself. This gave me instant positive results and ensured that the work flowed smoother.

Soft and smooth music was implemented in my office, home and car. Clients and friends visiting noticed immediately.

Most gave me good compliments for the choice of music. Music had always been one of my favorite past times. Therefore, this was not a chore to transition to more soft and smooth music. Simply listening to music was not all that I did. Music had to have meaning to me before I chose it. If the music included singing, I made sure that the words meant something to me and the listener. This became my trademark and I was always anxious to showoff my music collection. This collection included basically three types of music including smooth jazz.

Firmly I believed you put stress on yourself in most situations. Others don't cause you stress unless you allow them to. It was my belief that your decision to be with others, or do things you really don't want to was your personal choice. Further, I decided you don't always have to rush to accomplish personal or business tasks. Better organization and different approaches to situations or tasks became a main focus point for me. This plan of attack became a daily function and worked. No, I didn't become more robotic but writing things down in a more clear, concise and systematic fashion helped immensely.

The art of spacing things out became the norm not the exception. In other words, personal appointments such as doctor visits, banking and similar financial matters, etc. were put into separate days depending on the travel distance and normal time taken for such an appointment. Rarely did I put two different doctor visits on the same day. If I had an emergency situation such as a car repair and a doctor visit I tried real hard to put them on two distinctly different days. Business dealings were dealt with in a similar manner. In most cases I found myself having been the problem in the past, over committing or overbooking.

The decision to stick to my plans became more imminent and meaningful for me. Realizing others plans sometimes didn't work for me was most difficult. This was because you faced the hurdle of either hurting someone's feelings, losing a friendship, or jolting a business relationship. This meant saying no several times. However, in most cases the challenge worked for me and the other party because of pre-planning and early communication.

Having someone to share moments is optimum. but I realized you can't let that overwhelm you. Whenever there were times I didn't have a relationship at hand, I learned to not force it. It was to learn to love yourself as the songwriter said and have fun yourself always. Relationships come by your way on their own by the way you carry yourself, that is your attitude. No moping around, slumping, no sad faces became my motto. Laughter and energy became my trademarks whenever someone saw me whether the first time or every time. These became natural.

On the other hand I found time alone sometimes gave me time to reenergize myself, organize my thoughts and time more wisely. It was amazing how this helped to be alone sometimes and put my time to good use. This happened periodically instead of worrying about company or companionship. You might say I achieved attaining that peace of mind I had always sought after. You know even when I thought I was alone I found that inner peace and spiritual wisdom taught me by my grandparents.

5

PROPER ATTITUDE IN ALL SITUATIONS

When I grew up with my grandparents in Dawson, Georgia, I really did not know the meaning of attitude as people express it today. More importantly to me each day was doing the right things each day and going about my work and play joyously. My grandparents set the standards high for me but I didn't understand it while growing up. They never expressed disappointment, failure, nor worry in front of me.

Mama and Papa Charlie often used a word I learned to echo, sacrifice. Often I heard them used this word in cautions and chastisement to me. Phrases were used such as "boy, you've got to always sacrifice to have something. Boy, you don't know how we have sacrificed for you." These words did very little for me while growing up as a young boy but caused me to be fearful of when I heard the word sacrifice. It usually meant a whipping was coming if I kept going the same way after being cautioned by them more than once.

Sacrifice eventually became one of my most often used words to my children and to young people I mentored in youth sports and church. It meant being close to Christ to me. My approach to most things was Christ like, putting yourself last and other people ahead of yourself. After all it contained most of the word sacred in its spelling. Later I learned to use it synonymous to what ministers say "sowing seeds". This word helped shaped my attitude.

My life growing up was not living in desperation nor having unrealistic dreams. Life was always full of hope for every opportunity presented. These people treasured life and loved God. Often, both would say, always hold your head high and smile. That way people don't know whether or not you have something.

Their comments were brought to light when one of my middle school teachers used me as an example in defining the word haughty. Her comments to the class were "Joseph is haughty, look how proud he walks with his head high up in the air." How little they all knew where that attitude came from.

Understanding how they made ends meet financially and take care of me amazed me. Oftentimes I have reflected on times with them as I faced challenges alone or with my children. In each moment of reflection, I came out of it with a strong sense of security. Having observed them and the way they conducted themselves, their business dealings, their day to day lifestyles and their attitude toward people and life are excerpts of Christ stories in the bible.

Remember, we lived in a subsidized housing project. As I eventually understood it, subsidized meant low income people were eligible to pay low rent and the government paid a portion of the rent to a housing authority. Therefore, we were classified as poor to most people living outside of the housing project. Most of my friends whom I met through church or school lived outside of the project. Therefore, we were limited to our visitations to see each other. You've got to understand that these visitations were unilateral, that is, I always had to make the trip to my friends' houses when their parents allowed. This equaled to an average of two Sundays per month after church even during the summer months when school was out.

It never occurred to me that we were considered poor by most people around the city while growing up. My grandparents had firmly planted such a huge platform for me to live on. Their lifestyle was completely Christ centered but in 100 % exemplary fashion. They were not people who went to the streets to tell about their belief in Christ. You only heard about Christ loudly when a discussion was started by someone else. Their teachings to me were always wisdom filled and included biblical based backup if needed. We never argued the bible, their rock solid rule.

Their attitude toward Christ and life firmly cemented my course of life. Always be thankful for what you got was an expression that rang in my head until I left for college. That didn't mean accept life's setbacks and stay stuck in one place, they were quick to point out. That meant accept life's challenges and offerings as Christ presentments. These presentments most of the times were Christ's opportunities for you to do something with them. Many writers have said turn a negative into a positive.

My grandparents instilled in me an attitude to be appreciative of everything given to me. Always be positively vocal to the person or persons doing the giving. Most importantly give thanks to God. These sort of comments were always ended with the phrase, don't just settle. Keep working to make it better for yourself.

As a young college student I firmly grasped the meaning of attitude as a state of mind. This state of mind meant positive or negative to me. There was no in between or grey area. Therefore, I always pursued every challenge with 100 percent energy and a no failure approach. This always meant going extra miles to achieve desired results. This even existed in pursuing relationships with the opposite sex. If I wanted something bad enough persistence never caught me short.

Choosing a major in college was my first challenge. My precollege education and counselors suggested that I should go into the sciences because I had clearly demonstrated a love and knowledge for the sciences and math. When I arrived at college I had the idea that I should major in chemistry but I did not know how to choose a curriculum nor plan to use this type of degree after college. Further I did not know how to pursue education past undergraduate. My mission became to graduate from undergraduate school and choose a major to specialize in a major that helped people. These efforts sounded easy to achieve but it was mind boggling until late my freshman year. Having worked on campus in a work-study program meant I had an employment w-2 to file for income taxes. Most of the people I began to associate with had similar issues with this w-2 form. We all listened to one person who told us to go to a certain accounting professor who was helping all students who planned to pursue business related degrees.

Happily, I marched over to the Accounting department after getting directions to the location. After meeting this professor, he explained the process and proceeded to collect my work. He told me after collecting my work when to come back the next day and pick up my return since my return was so easy. When I got back with him, his words never left my mind, "look, never ask anyone else to do your return. You can do this yourself." He responded this way because of my many questions and I had given him the correct refund amounts of both federal and state returns before he finished

Needless to say, I chose to pursue a business administration degree. However, this same professor took me to the head of the business department who convinced me to specialize in accounting and choose business administration as a minor. This became my career path.

After progressing through my first two years of the program the department head had set for me, I became totally bonded with my career path. The department head always set challenges and goals for me. Each hurdle, I accepted and gave it 100% to master it. This grasped his attention as well as other professors and some students noticed my attitude. Gladly I accepted this professor's challenges on most tough assignments.

While in school, opportunities came my way such as summer jobs in my major field and part time jobs during school. Most of the time a professor in the department was instrumental in steering the assignment my way. Along with the job assignments came knowledge of how to pursue job opportunities in and after school.

One of my most memorable assignments was a program sponsored by the IRS during my junior year. The department head had provided a forum for the IRS to teach some students from our class at MBC, other AUC school students, and most Atlanta area colleges. During the second semester of the class, students were assigned to various Atlanta sites to do volunteer income tax work for people in the community. This program later became known as VITA.

Shortly after this assignment some of the students and myself became known to some local practicing accountants. These accountants hired us during income tax season and paid us decent wages based on our output. This was challenging, rewarding and grew our knowledge of taxation as well as the business community. This opportunity showed me entrepreneurial opportunities for the future. However, I knew experience was needed long before trials of any sort.

Therefore, I immediately focused on getting a job with a large company at the suggestion of the department head. He encouraged my graduating class and myself by assisting us with the interview process through these companies. His goals reached near and far. After trying his methods and using an attitude of gratitude from him, interviews were arranged in such cities as Atlanta, Chicago, Minnesota, and Baltimore. Offers were extended by the IRS, Baltimore and Georgia—Pacific, Portland, Oregon.

You guessed it. There was a major obstacle in my way. During my last collegiate year I had met the woman of my dreams in Atlanta and I did not want to leave her behind. Her tears as I embraced the Baltimore position caused me to reluctantly turn it down.

This created a huge new challenge. Where was I going to find gainful employment paying me the sort of wages companies outside of Atlanta were offering? After all, Atlanta's wages were well below the rest of the country's job market we had been warned as promising young collegiate graduates. Attitude and persistence didn't deter me. Proceeding on, I continued my job search with big companies in Atlanta. The search began in the local newspaper and I quickly landed a job with such a giant. This giant I'll leave anonymous because of its prominence in the workplace. This job paid okay but did not provide enough comfort for me to start a young family. The girl of my dreams and I had already decided we wanted a family right away.

My job search continued while I was in this giant's employ and I quickly landed a second job with a Pittsburgh based giant. That job appeared attractive enough for me to get in and start a family happily. The company took me in and provided sixteen successful years of employment. It provided a client base where I traveled, expenses paid by them and a company car. Most importantly I helped people in six states as a major lending source in six different job positions. Yes, I started and grew a family while employed by this giant.

Shortly before this giant sold most of its operations, I stepped out on faith on my own. Let me back up. It didn't quite happen that way. A continuing urge from God through the use of the Holy Spirit pushed me out of the door of this giant. This sent me to work in my own business as God had planned. The company didn't fire me nor ask me to leave but God would not peacefully let me stay any longer.

Like Moses, I had every excuse imaginable to God including I was not prepared financially. God didn't listen. He yanked me out of the door during the beginning of the income tax season of that year, never to look back or second guess him. Each day's approach took the right attitude but it worked using God's approach, pray without ceasing and keep your hands in God's hands as my grandparents instructed me. You know my professors and mentors along the way used the same techniques that my grandparents taught me.

6

TRUSTING IN GOD

As a young boy, my faith was firmly built on a foundation of trusting in God. Mama and Papa Charlie taught me to pray before making any major decision. When I deviated away from their teachings and did what I thought was right instead, uncertainty, frustration and disappointment often were the end results. Mama and Papa Charlie would often say, now are you ready to try things our way.

Our family home was in a local housing project with a fenced backyard. After my arrival in Atlanta several years ago, I met and heard several people from different other national cities who had lived in housing projects while growing up say housing projects were different when they grew up. They meant different in the sense that people lived in those projects and treated the premises as their own by keeping things clean and in order. This was definitely the case of our community housing project. People even respected each other and my grandparents were held in high regards by the project residents as well as residents in other neighborhoods in the small town. It always appeared that some of the biggest and roughest bullies had to come by my unit to live. You could hear them using profanity from several units away but as they neared our unit, they softly would say, keep it down, that's Mrs. Essie Mae's and Mr. Dave's house. Also, I remembered every week Mama had my first cousin and I mop the tile floors with pine sol-texize. The smell lasted a week.

Mama and Papa Charlie taught me well and showed me how to grow vegetables as well as plant fruit trees. In our vegetable garden were vegetables such as corn, tomatoes, onions, pepper, collards, turnips and okra. We had just enough room for a plum tree that spread so big that it grew as tall as the project unit and rested its branches on the roof.

Even though our space was limited Mama and Papa Charlie taught me how to maximize every inch of available space. Faith and patience were always needed each year to see if what you planted was going to come up and when. The fruit from the plum tree and vegetables from the garden were always good every year. We always had enough to share with neighbors and family members who visited. The plum tree became so famous and produced such big fruit that the neighborhood children would plan night raids from the roof of the housing unit. The tree's base was near the window of my grandparents' bedroom. Many times these raids were not successful as a result.

Mama had two younger sisters who lived in the same city but lived in their homes they owned. Each grew big gardens on their land near their homes. They always had me come over during the growing season and help them work their gardens. This meant using manual tools. They always had to uproot the soil neatly and in rows for planting. It also meant gathering the crops as they ripened. Both seemed equally hard to do because these sisters always got the most out of me. These sisters seemed to grow everything we didn't grow at our limited space housing project unit. They even grew big fruit and nut trees. Included were figs, peaches, plums and pecans. Their vegetable gardens were sprawling and had every vegetable imagined. Faith in God and patience persisted in everything these sisters did. As a result they were always rewarded. Even their pecan trees yielded enough pecans each year that they looked forward to paying their annual property tax bills.

These sisters would pay me every Saturday and sternly directed me to always go to my favorite department clothing store and buy clothing. The directive was always buy something every week to reward yourself even if it was just a tie clamp, tie, or pair of socks. When I needed to make a big purchase, such as a sports coat or suit, one of these Aunts would always go with me and make sure everything was color coordinated and fit properly. These sisters dressed pretty sharp themselves so I knew to obey.

Working for my Aunts in this manner taught me the value of work and to seek other opportunities. Such an opportunity came to me my first summer of high school. My high school sponsored a program called the Neighborhood Youth Core which was underwritten by the Federal Government. The job included working in the two city housing projects under a foreman. Ironically, my best friend (Marvin) and I got the job in the same two housing projects working with each other daily. My friend lived over ten miles away from my housing project with his parents in their home near the church we both attended regularly.

Marvin and I met the foreman and we both liked him and the description of the job. This foreman stood six feet five inches tall and was the Father/Great Grandfather of two eventual NBA talents. He gave us the descriptions of the job as general maintenance. General maintenance included laying tile, painting vacant units, light plumbing, small appliance repair, and yard work We soon found our niche as painters. The foreman saw this and placed us in every painting vacancy that came available. There was no idle time. Instead, the foreman would fill in trips between both housing projects with other tasks such as yard work.

This was a good summer job that lasted all summer. Marvin and I opted to work summers as long as the program lasted. The money was good and quickly showed both of us good working habits and ethics. Marvin's parents were equally as excited as my grandparents and Aunts were of both of us sticking it out as we did. They all knew we had a lot in common but working as long as we did surprised them all.

Marvin and I were classmates in high school, attended the same A.M.E. church and liked basketball a great deal. He and I played sandlot basketball regularly together but Marvin's older brother could play in a league with the other giants of our hometown. Marvin's older brother even played on the same collegiate team as one of the six Jones brothers who all played pro basketball. This was done while under basketball scholarship. Marvin and I lost regular contact with each other as I went away out of town to college to pursue a business degree. During some of my recent visits to relatives I learned that Marvin had become widely acclaimed as one of the top ministers in the local area of my hometown.

As I grew older my thirst for more work at higher wages grew. Entrepreneur work projects including yard work, telephone answering at a local funeral home and panting work resulted. All turned out to be successful ventures and made me enough money to start a small savings account and buy clothes. Mama saw this and gave me a smile of encouragement in her usual manner when I appeared on course to her. This became fun for both money and work. Even though my grandfather had died near the end of my freshman year, he had laid the blueprint for me and mama to follow. Those sisters of mama were always nearby if there ever appeared any uncertainty..

Mama taught me to pray every day and never let my faith in God waiver. God was the key to all things and you never would get anywhere without God, she constantly reminded me. My faith had grown with every trial and tribulation I soon discovered. One of the most difficult decisions of my youth was having to make decision to leave home and go away to college. Mama made the decision for me by telling me to go on and do what God had intended for me to do. God had made a way for me to go to school by making it possible financially through undergraduate financial assistance for all undergraduate work, she preached. Believe me, I didn't argue. I left with my luggage, faith and Mama's words of encouragement through collegiate years through graduation.

Faith in God helped me to land a job right after college with a fortune 100 company and Mama lived to see me get it. She also lived to see me come through my hometown on more than one occasion in a company car auditing some of the businesses I grew up around, lived to see me marry and to see my first born son. Mama even came and stayed in Atlanta in one of the most exclusive hotels that existed prior to her death. Through all of this faith grew and I knew Mama had passed the torch of faith to me to pass on to generations to come.

The Corporate world was a huge challenge but faith in God carried me mightily through six different successful managerial positions with the same company. Mama's teachings through examples showed me never stay at a place too long. She always said, son, don't get put out, leave on your own terms. This simply meant plan you exit. I did just that.

After sixteen years of service, I decided to take my part-time tax/bookkeeping practice to a full time level. No where near enough money was put aside in savings nor any place to realistic start this business full-time especially with a young family of four. However, God pulled me out of the door of Corporate America never to look back. Having left this company a year, several of the people from my old company called me and let me know that the company had dissolved and given everyone severance packages. Further reading showed me that this large company had dissolved by selling bits and pieces of the company to several other giant companies.

The Corporate world positions were mammoth hurdles for me. Nothing compared to running your own shop. At the same time, nothing could be more rewarding than enjoying your successes as your own operation moves on successfully. People have often asked me, if you had to do it all over again, would I trade places or change the way I did things? My answer was always no, I wouldn't change a thing. Every experience taught me an invaluable lesson. That produced wisdom.

Belief in God led me to find a remedy to better live with m.s. with no flare ups. God's way of living has kept me disease free from multiple sclerosis and all other diseases. My search led me to listen to statements from a medical doctor on national television. After listening to this doctor the first time, Dr. Lorraine Day, I could not believe that I heard a licensed medical doctor express belief in God and give full credit to God for curing her of breast cancer. Shortly after hearing her on television for the first time, I raced to purchase three different sets of Dr. Day's videos and her book. After fully reading the book and examining the tapes, I passed these on to friends and relatives with degenerative diseases. However, Dr. Day's work sent me in several directions for more research to support her findings and search answers to multiple sclerosis. Dr. Day's approach certainly sounded like an extension of the Holy Spirit talking to me as I took each step in faith.

Immediately after trying some of Dr. Day's and my own research strategies, I saw and felt improved changes. My research took on the same character as my childhood teachings and formal training in Corporate America. Determination showed me where there was a will there was a way. The most convincing indications of positive progress were my improved digestive system functions. My walking improvement followed nearly ninety days later. Approximately six months into trying a natural approach to improving my health I received improved medical opinions from two leading medical doctors, my regular urologist and my regular ophthalmologist.

This let me know not only had God stepped in but he had given me a message to keep on pursuing more of the research items to further improve and stay disease free. This message from God let me know I must share these miracles with others to help them improve. Further God let me know that Mama and Papa Charlie had instilled in me unwavering faith. It was years after Mama's death that I realized together they had given me the heart of a lion to venture through all challenges. They also gave me the courage of little David to pursue big victories but yet the spirit of God to remain humble in all dealings. Later I realized that people called this a gift from God. Often I have reminisced how I longed to have the same traits as I saw them exhibit. Thanks be to God.

7

MY LIFE WITH M.S. NOW

My life with m.s. now is best characterized as peaceful, energetic, healthy and happy. Finding the daily solutions I've outlined in the first six chapters of this book gave me the ingredients to a better quality of life. Life today is fruitful and eventful. Each day causes me to pause and give thanks to God as often as I can. Sometimes it is twice per day but more often it is more than twice per day.

Each early morning as I arise, I reflect back to the early challenging years of m.s.. This happens because I am so excited to be able to get up, read a short passage of scripture and get to walking each day before I start my full range of activities. Some days I miss reading my scripture early. When this happens usually an alarm goes off in my head later that day telling me that I failed to perform an invaluable duty of the day, give thanks to the lord for being able to look forward to doing the things I thought by now I could no longer do.

As I think back to the early years of m.s., I often wondered from day to day whether or not I would be able to walk on my own or be confined to a wheel chair. Walking meant inside of my home or outside to get in the car on my own, taking a leisurely stroll on a neighborhood sidewalk, strolling through a park holding my mates hand, walking on a golf course fairway or green, walking up or down stairs to a gym event, get out of the car to go inside of a bank or restaurant and getting out of the car to go inside of a mall. This concerned me the most about m.s. because this was the most pronounced effect m.s. visually had on me, limiting my walking ability and range of motion.

M.S. before my rehab period with Walt saw me stumbling and even falling in front of people. No matter how hard I tried this would stop for a short period and occur later. Denial set in and I couldn't accept these falls and stumbling as reality initially. Rehab with Walt helped but my post rehab work miraculously stopped most of this. Rarely, I see myself stumble and it is usually after some obstacle is in front of me that would normally cause anyone person to stumble. However, I'm conscious of the past problems so I maintain a step routine as part of my exercise routine three to four days per week.

Now I am better able to perform walking chores and the things above than I was prior to my extended rehab period. My morning walk is never less than three fourth mile per day without the thought of any kind of assistance. My walking is no longer cautious or tentative when I do my morning walk.

The walk is not as brisk as it once was before m.s. but it is comforting and mentally rewarding each morning to be able to walk when I once thought I would no longer be able to do this. This morning walk is in addition to all other daily aspects I've shared in this book. On my gym days, I still maintain my walk prior to going to the gym.

Flexibility plays its role in my daily life and in my maintenance of myself. At times I encounter a laundry list from my mate or client requests dictate that I perform some earlier than normal activities. When this happens I look at changing my walk times to mid day or late p.m. but the key is as my female gym partners say, "get it in." Excuses and change never stop me from maintaining myself daily. I live by a daily premise; excuses only satisfy those who make them. You make time for things that put your life in perspective.

Prior to my extended rehab period, attempting to take a daily morning walk was scary. Each day I approached lunch hours in those days with fear of leaving the office. In those days I always cheered for someone to volunteer to go get lunch for the staff and I. Today I look forward to my every morning walk, rain or shine. Most days I go get lunch unless someone is already headed in that direction. Some days a staff member and I go to lunch together now.

Exercise (weight resistance training) is minimum three days per week. Usually, I get in four days per week but never less than three days per week. This is not a chore. Instead, it remains challenging and rewarding to accomplish this standard I've set for myself. During my rehab training with Walt, he trusted me to do a run/walk routine on the three every other days I was not with him. Running ceased early in my rehab work with Walt because I was fearful of falling and injuring myself. However, walking was always done. Stumbling improved with the treatments Walt gave me and the biking.

Now, I perform what I term a bike/walk routine. My walk consists of three fourth mile and a stationary bike ride on the same day consists of no less than ten minutes. This routine adds flexibility to my total body movement and walking ability. Rare stumbling occurs daily.

Needless to say, it is gratifying to get the many compliments from the many people who see my physical conditioning and physique. This includes men and women of all ages. Many compliments come from the opposite sex who are years younger. This is a constant reminder that that the compliments are real. Also, it is soothing to the ego when the opposite sex compliments you daily. My favorite test is to meet eyes with a beautiful woman who takes a second look or third stare at you when she moves a way. This look or stare is not to be seen by me of course but my mannerism has become to look away after the first stare and look back at the person staring shortly afterwards.

Nutrition remains vitally important to me daily. My approach remains rigid in most areas. Particularly, food intake is cautious but continuing research and reading well documented and leading health authorities continue to show me that my changed nutritional habits play a key role in my continuing improved and good health. Later at the end of this section you will be able to compare my marginal changes to some added foods versus what I ate during the post rehab period.

Nutritionist Lindbergh was one of the many people of whom I used material during my search for answers to my illness and how to get better. Nutritionist Lindbergh's definition of degenerative disease painted a fascinating picture in my life during my post rehab years. Again she said that "degenerative diseases are not caused by viruses, bacteria, or parasites but the real killer is malnutrition, the absence of some substance (vitamin, mineral or trace element." Her comments spring boarded me into maintaining the sort of action I had already begun utilizing with my nutritional habits and search for even more knowledge.

It has been brought to my attention on numerous occasions during research that too little or too much of something causes problems. Always, this mystery sat before me with each nutritional trial. Reading with understanding and trusting God provided a solid base. But remember I maintained regular six month medical doctor visits to gauge my progress. No doctor was told what I was doing.

Today, I continue my yearning for knowledge by reading or listening to every echo or article I run across on the subject of nutritional habits. My brother-in-law always told me as a young adult, "Knowledge is power. You don't know how powerful you are. You will understand one day."

My liquid intake has been modified significantly as to the number of glasses of intake daily. Water remains between five to seven and one half eight ounce glasses daily. Juices have been cut back to three to five eight ounce glasses per day. The interval intake remains thirty minutes after drinking and one hour after eating before I consume more. This works well with my digestive system. After receiving a few cheap shot negative comments about my methods of eating and drinking, I learned to keep my comments about nutrition private. This works well and avoids arguments. After all I'm no doctor nor nutritionist.

Eating out remains secondary but I have select spots that I frequent when I do eat out. Usually, eating out consists mainly of vegetable plates where the establishments cook with non pork or beef products in their preparation process. Traveling long distances is very difficult. Short distances allow me to carry a bucket of ice to pack juices and certain vegetable items, mainly salads. The ice is replenished during the trip. Long distance and short distance traveling require a great deal of planning and organization prior to each trip. This area is still my most fearful and targeted area for improvement, traveling readiness.

A sample menu list of my food and liquid intake after my extended rehab period follows this write up.

Today I live on top of a hill overlooking cars, the neighborhood pool, other housing units, and sites. I can see all people around me but they may not see me.

When I grew up with my grandmother, Essie Mae and grandfather, Dave, we, lived at the back of a housing project. Our unit was in a section that was at the bottom of a hill. We played basketball on that hill and it was a favorite fun time spot for me and the other project children. The neighborhood pool and mobile library drop off port were nearby and adjacent to the final section of the housing project units. Views from the hill were often cloudy because of the dust caused by the nearby peanut mill.

Now if I choose I can walk down the hill I live on to the pool. But most of time I enjoy the views and air surrounding me from my patio on top of the hill.

Today my optimum daily number of sleep hours is 7.5 hours. Regularly, I get 6.5 hours to seven hours of sleep per night. The optimum number, 7.5 hours is reached two to three nights per week. Some weeknights I get a full eight hours per night of sleep. This happens about two nights per week. Rarely do I exceed eight hours of sleep per night.

Every day sleep is critical to my ability to function at peak performance. When I awake each day I feel totally refreshed from the previous day. There are no side effects, no hangovers, no aches nor pains, just plain refreshed. It is a feeling of ready to go and rejuvenation.

The partner to sleep, rest, has become my sidekick. Everyday I take one and one half to two hours of rest. This is time I spend doing nothing including thinking about nothing.

Today I continue to stay away from stress filled events. This includes careful scrutiny of my television viewing. Most funerals I send flowers. Occasionally, I attend funerals. It's not even a second thought to decline an offer for an engagement if I have already planned something.

Now I attend more later evening outside functions when invited. This is still carefully planned and I don't overdo it. Sporting and entertainment events are back on my agenda but in moderation.

Medications for m.s. and other degenerative conditions are non existent for me today. What a joy it is to not worry about side effects and sleepless nights.

Maintaining a positive attitude and trusting in God daily are required, not options.

Menus-M.S. now

Breakfast list

Strawberries
Large bowl grapes
One whole banana
Sliced apples
Sliced cantaloupe during season, sliced melons during season
1 peach during season
Large bowl oatmeal
Smoothie (breakfast meal itself) 100 % whole honey
wheat rolls

Combinations of most of the above fruits are eaten every breakfast. Grapes and oatmeal are rarely absent from a breakfast meal. A smoothie is substituted as a meal rarely one day of the week.

Lunch

Vegetarian plate consisting of any combination of the following vegetables
Collards
Turnips
Corn boiled on the cob or cream style
Green beans
Lima beans
Carrot soufflé
Yams

Sliced tomatoes
Occasional okra with tomato and corn mixed, broccoli
Carrots
Peas green or black eyed
Baked potato
Corn bread muffins
Or corn bread sticks
Or whole wheat dinner rolls
Brown rice
Added to any of the above vegetables certain days that I don't eat a vegetarian plate are
Grilled wild salmon two to three days per week
Grilled wild talapia or wild tuna once per week

Any combinations of the above vegetables are used but never rice with a green leafy vegetable. I always eat a green leafy vegetable each day for lunch

Dinner

Fruit medley (once per every two weeks)
Tuna submarine sandwich (no more than twice per week)
Grilled salmon (once to twice per week)
Baked fish (usually tilapia)
Baked potato
Boiled corn on the cob
Potato chips (baked)
Broccoli (steamed)
Carrots (steamed)
Rice

Sliced tomato
Vegetable garden salad, usually spinach or lettuce with tomatoes and health food selected salad dressing. Whole wheat dinner rolls

Daily liquid intake

Early a.m., one glass water
Following the water no less than thirty minutes, one glass of
100% orange juice

Breakfast

No less than one hour after breakfast, one glass of either 100%
Carrot juice or 100% apple-carrot juice
No less than thirty minutes after last juice 1 glass of green leafy
vegetable juice with barley included.

Lunch

One hour after lunch, more juice usually 100% tomato juice
or carrot juice
For next few hours after waiting thirty minutes apart I continue juicing and some water mixed in between.
Juices are 100% carrot, apple carrot or green leafy vegetable
juice with barley included.

Dinner

One glass water

No more than five glasses of 100% juice is drank per day.

RECOMMENDED READING LIST

Dr. Rho's Ten Secrets to Living Healthy, Rovenia M. Brock, Ph. D.

How To Be Your Own Nutritonist, Dr. Stuart Berger, M.D.

Eat To Live, Joel Fuhrman, M.D.

Secrets Of Sleep, Alexander Borbely

Your Best Life Now, Joel Osteen

Health Walk, Bob Carlson & O.J. Seiden, M.D.

Walking Medicine, Gary Yanker & Kathy Burton

Miracle Cures From The Bible, Reese Dublin

Getting Started On Getting Well, Lorraine Day, M.D.

Take Charge of Your Health, Gladys Lindberg and Judy Lindberg Mcfarland

978-0-595-44419-9
0-595-44419-9

Printed in the United States
By Bookmasters